PARKINSON'S DISEASE DIET COOKBOOOK FOR BEGINNERS

A Complete Guide To Managing Your Symptoms Through Nutrition: 150+ Recipes | 28-Day Meal Plan

JESSICA C. STEPHEN

DISCLAIMER

The information in this book is meant solely for educational reasons. This book's contents are not meant to be used in place of expert medical advice, diagnosis, or treatment. Any decisions you make about your health must be discussed with a licensed healthcare provider.

Every effort has been made by the author to guarantee that the material in this book is correct and current as of the date of publication. Still, since medical knowledge advances rapidly, new studies might be conducted that change our understanding this illness and how best to manage it with food.

This book may contains references to and mentions of various people, things, websites, organizations, and other entities that the author does not support, advocate, or have any association with. There is no implied sponsorship or collaboration; all references and remarks are made only for informational purposes.

In order to address their individual health concerns, readers are advised to independently verify any information contained in this book and to consult with healthcare specialists. Any negative effects arising from the use or implementation of the material in this book, whether direct or indirect, are not the responsibility of the author or the publisher.

The dietary suggestions and counsel provided in this book are broad in scope and might not be appropriate for every individual. Readers are recommended to seek tailored counsel from trained healthcare specialists as individual health problems and demands differ.

The reader accepts the conditions of this disclaimer by reading this book.

FACTS ABOUT THIS BOOK

The book "Parkinson's Disease diet cookbook for beginners " is an extensive and priceless tool for everyone with Parkinson's disease, as well as caretakers and medical experts. Seeing how important it is to comprehend Parkinson's disease from all angles, the first few chapters offer a comprehensive overview of the illness. The book dives deeply into the complexities of the illness, looking at risk factors, symptoms, causes, and the state of current treatments as well as their drawbacks. The reader's understanding of the complex connection between diet and Parkinson's disease is established by this core knowledge.

The next chapters emphasize the role that nutrition plays in the management of Parkinson's disease. The book covers dietary inadequacies frequently linked to Parkinson's disease and clarifies the critical role that nutrition plays in maintaining brain function. The book's practical method for putting dietary changes into practice is one of its strongest points. A balanced diet, emphasis on key nutrients, and suggestions for certain foods and food groups are all covered in the section on developing a Parkinson 's-friendly diet. A practical layer is added by taking dietary limitations into account, which guarantees that readers can customize their diets to meet their specific needs.

Examining the relationship between medicine and diet is one of the book's standout aspects. An in-depth discussion of the relationship between nutrition and Parkinson's medication is covered in Chapter 4, along with suggestions for when to eat and how to adapt to adverse effects. This sophisticated method recognizes the relationship between diet and medicine, which is an important but sometimes disregarded factor in Parkinson's disease management.

Additionally, the book addresses particular symptoms related to Parkinson's disease, going beyond basic dietary recommendations. Nutritional options for symptom management include chapters that explore dietary ways to improve digestive health, cognitive function, and motor complaints. With well-informed food decisions, readers are empowered to proactively control their symptoms thanks to this specific instruction.

Other important facets of health that are covered in the book include weight control, staying hydrated, and learning about unique diets like the Mediterranean and ketogenic diets. The book helps readers to make well-informed judgments on supplementary methods to their nutritional regimen by offering evidence-based information about supplements and their potential advantages and risks.

There are chapters devoted to food preparation advice specifically for Parkinson's patients, demonstrating that practical factors are not disregarded. Convenience and nutrition are balanced by using flexible cooking methods, simple-to-chew recipes, and meal-planning tools.

The book acknowledges that lifestyle factors that go beyond nutrition play a role in Parkinson's disease. It offers a comprehensive viewpoint on well-being by addressing the effects of exercise, stress reduction, and good sleep hygiene. The necessity of a multidisciplinary strategy incorporating nutritionists and healthcare professionals is highlighted by the final point, which highlights the significance of overcoming obstacles and seeking professional help.

"Parkinson's Disease Nutrition" essentially acts as a thorough manual that bridges the knowledge gap between theory and actual application. It provides the information and resources required for people with Parkinson's disease, their carers, and medical professionals to understand the intricate relationship between nutrition and the disease.

TABLE OF CONTENTS

CHAPTER 12   52

28-DAY MEAL PLAN   56

CHAPTER 1

AN OVERVIEW OF PARKINSON'S ILLNESS

A Brief Overview of Parkinson's Disease

Movement is the main symptom of Parkinson's disease (PD), a neurological condition that progresses over time. The substantianigra, a part of the brain in charge of motor function, exhibits a progressive degeneration of dopamine-producing neurons. A neurotransmitter called dopamine is essential for directing steady, fluid muscular actions. A variety of motor and non-motor symptoms that accompany the degeneration of these neurons severely impair the quality of life for people with Parkinson's disease.

Although cases with early start are possible, Parkinson's disease usually presents in people over 60. Although genetics may be involved in certain cases, the majority of PD cases are thought to be sporadic, and the precise origin of the disease is still unknown. Lewy bodies, and aberrant protein deposits in the brain that contribute to neuronal degeneration, are the characteristic pathogenic features of Parkinson's disease.

Factors at Risk and Causes

Parkinson's disease has a complex and multifaceted precise etiology. In some circumstances, heredity is a part, but environmental variables also matter a lot. There is evidence linking an elevated risk of Parkinson's disease to exposure to specific chemicals, including pesticides and herbicides. Head injuries and a medical history of specific illnesses may further increase the risk.

The main risk factor for Parkinson's disease is age, as the disease is more common in those who are older. Men are typically more susceptible than women, thus there are gender disparities as well. Furthermore, a new study indicates that Parkinson's disease may be influenced by the gastrointestinal tract and that the gut-brain axis may contribute to the onset of the condition.

Signs And Advancement

A variety of motor and non-motor symptoms, varying in severity from person to person, are present with Parkinson's disease. Postural instability, stiffness, bradykinesia (slowed movements), and tremors are examples of motor symptoms. Mood problems, autonomic dysfunction, sleep abnormalities, and cognitive impairment are examples of non-motor symptoms.

Parkinson's disease progresses gradually and may take years to fully manifest. Early signs could include a minor limp or tremors, but as the illness progresses, symptoms get worse and can cause serious disability. The impact on routine activities like dressing and walking gets harder to handle. Later stages of the disease may also cause cognitive impairment, including dementia, which would make treatment even more difficult.

Present Interventions And Restrictions

Since treatment for Parkinson's disease is not yet available, management of the condition focuses on symptom relief. The main pharmacological strategy consists of drugs designed to either replicate or raise dopamine's actions in the brain. The mainstay of treatment is levodopa, which relieves motor symptoms and is a precursor to dopamine. Long-term usage, however, may result in side effects such as dyskinesias and motor irregularities.

However, pharmaceutical therapies come with drawbacks and their effectiveness may wane with time. Some patients with severe Parkinson's disease may benefit from surgical procedures like deep brain stimulation. Other important aspects of symptom management include physical therapy and lifestyle changes.

Even with these therapies, Parkinson's disease is still difficult to treat completely. The goal of ongoing research is to improve outcomes and quality of life for those afflicted with this devastating condition by exploring novel therapeutic options such as gene therapies and neuroprotective measures.

CHAPTER 2

Nutrition is Crucial for Parkinson's Disease Management

When it comes to treating Parkinson's disease, a progressive neurological disease that largely affects the motor system, nutrition is crucial. For those who have Parkinson's disease, a healthy diet is crucial since it can have a big impact on their quality of life and general health.

The treatment of motor symptoms, including bradykinesia, stiffness, and tremors, is one of the most important factors. Since some foods make it easier for Parkinson's treatments to be absorbed and used, eating a healthy diet can help maximize the effectiveness of prescribed medications. Sustaining a healthy diet can also help avoid issues arising from adverse drug reactions, like nausea or constipation.

Nutrition also helps to maintain muscle function and strength, which is important for people with Parkinson's disease because they frequently experience weakness and stiffness in their muscles. Maintaining muscular function and preventing malnutrition, which can worsen Parkinson's disease symptoms, requires a well-balanced diet with enough protein, vitamins, and minerals.

Keeping a healthy weight is also essential for controlling Parkinson's because being underweight or overweight might present difficulties. An inadequate diet helps avoid inadvertent weight loss, guaranteeing that people with

Parkinson's disease have the stamina and energy required for everyday tasks. In contrast, keeping a healthy weight can promote mobility and lessen joint tension.

Beyond the physical dimensions, Parkinson's patients' mental and cognitive health are impacted by their diet. It may be possible to improve cognitive function and possibly slow down the cognitive decline linked to Parkinson's disease by eating a balanced diet high in antioxidants, omega-3 fatty acids, and other neuroprotective nutrients.

How Diet Impacts Mental Health:

The relationship between diet and brain health is especially important when considering Parkinson's disease, which is defined by the progressive loss of dopaminergic neurons in the brain. In addition to affecting neurotransmitter synthesis and offering protection against oxidative stress, nutrients are essential for maintaining brain function overall.

The function of antioxidants, such as vitamins C and E, in reducing oxidative stress and inflammation in the brain, is one important component. An antioxidant-rich diet may help reduce oxidative stress, which may help delay the onset of Parkinson's disease. Oxidative stress is linked to the pathophysiology of Parkinson's disease.

Furthermore, an abundance of fatty fish, flaxseeds, and walnuts contain omega-3 fatty acids, which have been linked to cognitive health and may even have neuroprotective properties. These fats support the structural integrity of brain cell membranes and may regulate inflammatory processes, opening up a possible treatment option for Parkinson's disease-related cognitive impairment.

Micronutrients such as B vitamins—specifically, B6, B9 (folate), and B12—are necessary for the production of neurotransmitters, including dopamine, which is lacking in Parkinson's disease. It is essential to maintain healthy brain function and boost neurotransmitter generation by ensuring an appropriate intake of these vitamins through diet or supplementation.

Nutritional Inadequacies with Parkinson's Disease:

Parkinson's disease patients may experience severe symptom exacerbation and compromised general health as a result of nutritional deficits. One frequent worry is the possibility of malnutrition, which is frequently linked to issues like swallowing problems, decreased appetite, and adverse drug reactions. Parkinson's disease symptoms, both motor and non-motor, might get worse due to malnutrition, which can also cause weight loss, weariness, and muscle wasting.

Given that several Parkinson's disease treatments compete with dietary protein for absorption, there is a special emphasis on protein consumption in this context. To maximize the efficiency of medication and provide proper nutrition, it is often advised to balance protein intake throughout the day rather than consuming it at one meal.

Deficits in vitamins and minerals may also accelerate the development of Parkinson's disease. Low vitamin D, for example, has been linked to a higher risk of fractures and falls, which are major concerns for people with

Parkinson's disease because of their decreased mobility and balance. As a result, it's critical to maintain adequate levels of vitamin D through food and sun exposure.

Furthermore, deficits in B vitamins—particularly B12—can worsen neurological symptoms and affect cognitive performance. Parkinson's sufferers ought to keep an eye on their B vitamin levels and, should shortages be found, think about supplementing.

In summary, taking care of nutritional requirements is essential to the all-encompassing therapy of Parkinson's disease. An individualized and balanced diet can have a beneficial effect on managing symptoms, promoting brain health, and reducing the likelihood of nutritional deficiencies that could worsen the difficulties faced by Parkinson's patients. The quality of life for those with Parkinson's can be improved by using a comprehensive strategy that includes medicine, exercise, and a healthy diet.

CHAPTER 3

MAKING A DIET SUITABLE FOR PARKINSON'S

Creating an Equilibrium Diet for Individuals with Parkinson's Disease

To properly control their symptoms and preserve overall health, people with Parkinson's disease must eat a balanced diet. To supply vital vitamins, minerals, and antioxidants, it should consist of a range of nutrient-dense foods. Whole foods including fruits, vegetables, lean meats, and whole grains should be the main focus of attention. A wide range of nutrients included in these foods support general health.

Retaining a healthy weight is crucial for Parkinson's disease management and for enhancing mobility. By assisting in the attainment and maintenance of a healthy weight, a balanced diet lowers the risk of issues associated with undernutrition and obesity. Dehydration can worsen symptoms like weariness and constipation, so staying properly hydrated is also essential.

Walnuts, flaxseeds, and fatty fish are examples of foods high in omega-3 fatty acids that may also have neuroprotective properties. These good fats help the brain work better and might even slow down Parkinson's disease progression. In general, Parkinson's patients' well-being is greatly aided by a balanced diet that is customized to meet their unique needs and preferences.

Vital Elements for Individuals with Parkinson's Disease

A few key nutrients are essential for both promoting general health and controlling the symptoms of Parkinson's disease. Due to increased oxidative damage in the brain, antioxidants, which are contained in fruits and vegetables, help shield cells from oxidative stress. This is especially significant for people with Parkinson's disease. It is advised to get enough sunshine exposure or take supplements of vitamin D as it is crucial for bone health and may have neuroprotective benefits.

Parkinson's patients should take into account their protein intake because certain drugs may conflict with amino acids for absorption. Managing any possible drug interactions can be facilitated by distributing protein consumption throughout the day and selecting lean protein sources.

Some Parkinson's patients have increased homocysteine levels; B vitamins, especially B6 and B12, are essential for nerve function and may help lower these levels. Fortified meals, leafy greens, and whole grains are great providers of these vitamins.

Food Groups and Suggested Foods

Nutrient-dense foods that support general health and symptom management are the focus of a Parkinson's disease-friendly diet. Antioxidant-rich fruits and vegetables have to be a regular part of your diet. Because they may have neuroprotective effects, cruciferous vegetables, leafy greens, and berries are especially advantageous.

Whole grains include fiber and other nutrients. Examples of these are brown rice, quinoa, and oats. Lean protein foods, such as beans, tofu, fish, and fowl, maintain the health of muscles without interfering with prescription drugs.

Including omega-3 fatty acids in diets through foods like salmon, chia seeds, and flaxseeds may improve brain function. Parkinson's patients should make sure they are adequately hydrated throughout the day by drinking plenty of water.

Dietary Guidelines And Things To Keep In Mind

Parkinson's disease patients may need to think about making certain dietary adjustments and limits, even though there isn't a one-size-fits-all solution.

It is important to consider the potential interactions between medications and specific diets, especially those high in protein. Patients should collaborate closely with their medical team to figure out the best way to divide up their daily protein intake.

Sometimes certain drugs can interfere with the body's ability to absorb nutrients, necessitating the use of supplements. In particular, if people are not getting enough calcium and vitamin D from their food or exposure to sunlight, supplements may be advised to maintain bone health.

Furthermore, swallowing and chewing difficulties can affect some Parkinson's disease patients, making it difficult for them to eat specific types of food. Under such circumstances, it becomes imperative to alter the texture of foods or add nutrient-dense, readily digestible alternatives.

A customized approach to dietary limits and considerations is essential for enhancing the nutritional status and general well-being of people with Parkinson's disease, taking into account the possible effects of drugs, personal preferences, and any underlying health problems.

CHAPTER 4

Interaction Between Diet And Parkinson's Medicine

Medicines and diet must be carefully balanced in the therapy of Parkinson's disease since their interactions can greatly affect how well a patient responds to treatment. A major Parkinson's drug, levodopa competes with other amino acids in the small intestine for absorption and is a precursor to dopamine. Levodopa's effectiveness may be diminished as a result of this competition affecting its absorption. To minimize this, patients are frequently instructed to take levodopa empty-handed or in conjunction with a low-protein diet. Patients should carefully consider how much protein they eat since too much protein can affect how well levodopa is absorbed.

Furthermore, the metabolism of drugs might be affected by specific nutrients and dietary components. For example, levodopa's therapeutic effects may be lessened by vitamin B6, which is present in a variety of meals and can speed up the drug's breakdown. As such, people with Parkinson's disease should be aware of the nutrients they consume and collaborate closely with medical practitioners to modify their diet to maximize the effectiveness of their medications.

When To Take Medicine And Eat

A crucial part of controlling Parkinson's disease is scheduling meals and prescriptions. Parkinson's patients are frequently instructed to take their medications—especially levodopa—either empty-handed or with a low-protein diet. This is due to the possibility that protein will outcompete levodopa for absorption, lowering its potency. It is therefore recommended that patients carefully plan their medicine doses around meal times.

The time of meals is also very important since variations in blood sugar levels affect how well drugs are absorbed and how Parkinson's symptoms manifest. Frequent, balanced meals aid in the maintenance of stable blood sugar levels, avoiding swings that may impair the absorption of medications and general symptom management. To ensure the best possible therapeutic outcomes and symptom management throughout the day, people with Parkinson's disease must collaborate closely with their healthcare team to develop a regular meal and drug plan.

Adapting Diet To Adverse Drug Reactions

Parkinson's patients may need to modify their diet due to side effects from their meds. For instance, taking certain drugs may cause nausea or gastrointestinal problems. Under such circumstances, medical practitioners could suggest dietary adjustments, like smaller, more frequent meals or particular foods that are easier on the digestive tract. Choosing foods that are readily digested and drinking enough water can also be very important in minimizing adverse effects from medications.

Certain drugs may also be a factor in weight fluctuations. Healthcare professionals who work with patients who are losing weight might recommend calorie- and nutrient-dense foods to assist them in staying at a healthy weight. On the other hand, those who are gaining weight could require nutritional interventions that center on limiting portion sizes and selecting low-calorie alternatives.

In conclusion, managing Parkinson's disease holistically necessitates an awareness of the complex interactions that exist between dietary choices and pharmaceuticals. People with Parkinson's can maximize their general well-being and improve the efficacy of their treatment plan by carefully planning meals, taking into account potential food combinations, and modifying the diet to minimize drug side effects. A customized and successful dietary plan in the setting of Parkinson's disease requires regular discussion with medical professionals.

CHAPTER 5

DIETARY APPROACHES TO SYMPTOM CONTROL

<u>Using Diet To Treat Motor Symptoms</u>

The main motor signs of Parkinson's disease, a neurodegenerative condition, are tremors, bradykinesia, and postural instability. Dietary modifications can support traditional therapies, even though drugs are an essential part of controlling these symptoms. Maximizing the consumption of anti-inflammatory foods and antioxidants is one important dietary strategy. Certain substances can alleviate inflammation and oxidative stress, two factors linked to the advancement of Parkinson's disease.

Consuming an abundance of colorful fruits and vegetables, especially leafy greens and berries, will supply vital antioxidants like vitamin C and flavonoids. Flaxseeds and fatty fish are rich sources of omega-3 fatty acids, which have anti-inflammatory qualities and may also have neuroprotective effects. Additionally, levodopa-induced changes in reaction to medicine can be controlled by ensuring an adequate intake of protein, spread evenly throughout the day.

A typical Parkinson's drug called carbidopa-levodopa competes with several amino acids in the stomach for absorption. Thus, the best time to consume protein can improve the medication's effectiveness.

Furthermore, swallowing difficulties are a potential complication for some Parkinson's patients, which may result in insufficient nutritional intake.

These issues can be resolved with meals that have been texture-modified and adequate hydration, which guarantees enough nutrients without sacrificing safety.

Nutrition And Parkinson's Disease Cognitive Function

Nutritional techniques can help maintain cognitive function, which is important for those with Parkinson's disease who are at risk of cognitive damage. Crucial elements of a neuroprotective diet include antioxidants, omega-3 fatty acids, and B vitamins, which are important for brain function. Neurotransmitter synthesis and cognitive function depend on B vitamins, particularly B6, B12, and folate. Foods such as fish, leafy greens, legumes, and lean meats are good sources of these vitamins.

Antioxidants, such as vitamins C and E, aid in the fight against oxidative stress, a factor in cognitive impairment. Antioxidant-rich foods can be included in a regular diet. Examples of these foods include berries, citrus fruits, nuts, and seeds. Omega-3 fatty acids are mostly present in fatty fish, such as trout and salmon, and they may help Parkinson's patient's brain health in addition to having been linked to cognitive advantages.

Another crucial component of cognitive health is blood sugar regulation. A modest consumption of healthy fats and complex carbs, including those found in whole grains and legumes, can help control blood sugar levels and give the brain a constant supply of energy. Additionally, it's critical to drink enough water because dehydration can impair cognitive performance.

Enhanced Digestive Health

Constipation to problems with gastrointestinal motility are among the main symptoms of Parkinson's disease that are related to digestive issues. When it comes to treating these digestive issues, nutrition is crucial. To encourage regular bowel movements and avoid constipation, a sufficient intake of fiber is necessary. Good sources of fiber that can be incorporated into a daily diet are whole grains, fruits, vegetables, and legumes.

Parkinson's sufferers may also benefit from probiotics, which are good microorganisms that promote gut health. These beneficial microorganisms can enter the digestive system through fermented foods such as sauerkraut, kefir, yogurt, and others. Probiotics may help maintain the health of the gastrointestinal system generally and have been connected to increased gut motility.

Staying hydrated is essential for maintaining healthy digestive processes. Dehydration can exacerbate constipation and is a side effect of Parkinson's medicine and aging in general. Digestion problems can be mitigated by making sure you consume enough fluids, such as water, and hydrating foods like fruits and soups.

All things considered, a comprehensive dietary plan for controlling Parkinson's disease must include addressing motor symptoms with a neuroprotective diet, bolstering cognitive performance with nutrient-rich foods, and enhancing gut health with fiber and probiotics. Not only do these dietary therapies try to reduce symptoms, but they also improve the general health and quality of life for Parkinson's patients.

CHAPTER 6

HYDRATION AND PARKINSON'S

Importance of Hydration in Parkinson's

Drinking enough water is essential for good health, but for those who have Parkinson's disease, it's even more important because of the unique difficulties they must overcome. Parkinson's disease is a neurological condition that impairs movement and can cause a range of symptoms, both motor and non-motor. For people with Parkinson's disease, staying properly hydrated is crucial to their overall health because it can directly affect their cognitive and physical abilities.

Hydration is important for Parkinson's patients for several reasons, chief among which is that it may affect the efficacy of medications. Many people with Parkinson's disease depend on medications to control their symptoms, and drinking enough water can have an impact on how well these medications are absorbed and distributed throughout the body. Dehydration can worsen motor symptoms and lower the effectiveness of prescribed drugs, which can lower the patient's quality of life.

In addition, staying hydrated is crucial for preserving cognitive function. Cognitive impairment and confusion are common in people with Parkinson's disease, and dehydration can exacerbate these symptoms. Drinking enough water promotes healthy brain function and helps reduce some of the cognitive problems related to Parkinson's disease.

Additionally, staying hydrated helps to lessen Parkinson's non-motor symptoms like constipation. Smoother bowel motions are made possible by a well-hydrated digestive tract, which lessens the discomfort that Parkinson's sufferers often experience from constipation.

In conclusion, the significance of staying hydrated in Parkinson's disease extends beyond basic health concerns. The management of non-motor symptoms, cognitive function, and the efficacy of medications are all directly impacted by it, underscoring its crucial role in the comprehensive care of stroke victims.

Advice on Maintaining Hydration:

Many people struggle daily to stay properly hydrated, and people with Parkinson's disease may experience more difficulties because of the nature of their illness. But putting sensible measures into practice can make a big difference in sustaining appropriate water levels and promoting general well-being.

A useful piece of advice for those with Parkinson's disease is to develop a regimented water intake. Establishing regular intervals for drinking liquids during the day—for example, in between doses of medications or with meals—can promote constant hydration and help establish a habit.

Furthermore, hydration apps or water bottles with measured marks can be used as tools to track daily water intake and act as reminders.

Selecting the appropriate fluids is equally crucial. Although the main source of hydration is water, including meals high in water content, such as fruits and vegetables, can help increase total fluid intake. However, people should watch how much alcohol and caffeine they consume because these can have diuretic effects that raise the risk of fluid loss.

Another essential component of encouraging hydration in Parkinson's patients is environment adaptation. Independent and comfortable drinking can be promoted by making sure fluids are easily accessible, utilizing straw cups or other adaptive drinking aids, and removing any obstructions that can impede mobility.

Personalized hydration regimens require cooperation with medical professionals. Dietitians and medical professionals can provide customized advice depending on each person's needs, taking into account things like medication schedules, dietary restrictions, and particular Parkinson's disease symptoms.

Through the implementation of these suggestions into their daily routine, people with Parkinson's disease can improve their hydration habits, thereby addressing a critical component of their overall health management.

Dehydration's Effects on Parkinson's Symptoms

Dehydration can exacerbate problems that people with Parkinson's disease already encounter by having a significant impact on the disease's symptoms and course. Dehydration affects Parkinson's symptoms in more ways than only the physical discomfort of thirst. It affects both the motor and non-motor elements of the disease.

One important effect of dehydration is that it can reduce the effectiveness of Parkinson's disease treatments. Since many of these drugs are taken orally, dehydration may make it more difficult for the digestive system to absorb them. People may thus encounter variations in the management of their symptoms, such as worsening tremors, stiffness, and trouble moving around.

Another factor that exacerbates Parkinson's disease's non-motor symptoms is dehydration. Dehydration of the brain can worsen cognitive performance, which is already poor in Parkinson's disease patients. Increased confusion, focus issues, and a general deterioration in mental acuity may result from this.

Dehydration can make motor symptoms worse, like stiffness and cramping in the muscles. Maintaining muscular function and flexibility depends on adequate hydration, and people with Parkinson's disease may feel more uncomfortable and have restricted movement if they don't get enough fluids.

Furthermore, dehydration might exacerbate gastrointestinal problems like constipation which people with Parkinson's disease frequently have. Drinking enough water is essential for maintaining a healthy digestive system and avoiding issues brought on by bowel irregularity.

In conclusion, dehydration has a variety of consequences on Parkinson's symptoms, affecting both the disease's non-motor and motor components. For Parkinson's patients and their carers, understanding the relationship between hydration and symptom management is crucial, emphasizing the need to give proper fluid intake priority as part of an all-encompassing strategy for Parkinson's care.

CHAPTER 7

Variations In Weight In Parkinson's Disease

Patients with Parkinson's disease (PD) frequently experience fluctuations in their weight, which can have a substantial effect on their general health and well-being. Weight gain and loss are both possible in Parkinson's disease (PD), which poses a difficult task for both the affected person and their caregivers. Muscle tremors, dysphagia, and rigidity are all linked to weight loss because they might make it harder to chew and swallow food, which reduces food intake. Conversely, alterations in metabolism, side effects from medications, and a decrease in physical activity can all lead to weight gain.

Common motor symptoms of Parkinson's disease (PD) include tremors and muscle rigidity, which can increase energy expenditure and lead to inadvertent weight loss. Additionally, reduced food intake, malnutrition, and consequent weight loss can result from dysphagia, a difficulty with swallowing. On the other hand, some PD patients may gain weight as a result of their decreased physical activity levels brought on by their motor deficits. Weight fluctuations may also be influenced by medications used to treat Parkinson's disease symptoms; certain drugs may stimulate appetite, while others may have the reverse effect.

Techniques For Maintaining A Healthful Weight

It's critical to maintain a healthy weight when dealing with Parkinson's disease to preserve general health and properly manage symptoms. To address the several causes affecting weight changes in PD, a multifaceted approach is required. Exercise regimens customized to each person's skills can assist in increasing muscle strength, control metabolism, and offset the sedentary consequences of motor symptoms. Maintaining a healthy weight is facilitated by physical activity, which might also potentially mitigate certain non-motor symptoms linked to Parkinson's disease.

When it comes to controlling weight, dietary factors are crucial for people with Parkinson's disease. A nutrient-dense, well-balanced diet can boost energy levels, alleviate nutritional shortages, and promote general health. Consuming enough protein is especially crucial since it can support the maintenance of muscular mass and strength. To treat dysphagia and associated difficulties, speech and occupational therapy may help enable people to eat a varied and nourishing diet.

Handling Shifts In Appetite

Variations in appetite are a common aspect of Parkinson's disease and may be responsible for variations in weight. Maintaining ideal nutrition and quality of life requires an understanding of these changes and taking appropriate action. To treat medication-related changes in appetite, medication adjustments may be considered, under the supervision of a healthcare provider. Open communication regarding any changes in appetite is essential for patients with Parkinson's disease and their healthcare team, as this information can inform individualized interventions.

Non-pharmacological methods can be used in certain situations to treat changes in appetite. These could include eating smaller, more often meals, selecting foods high in nutrients, and drinking enough of water.

People who experience changes in their appetite can benefit from psychological support, such as counseling and mental health programs, which can help them manage the emotional components of these swings. Maintaining the best potential results for people with Parkinson's disease requires regular engagement with healthcare providers and regular monitoring of weight and nutritional condition. These factors allow for the adaptation of methods as the disease advances.

CHAPTER 8

PARKINSON'S DISEASE AND SPECIAL DIETS

Nutritional Benefits Of A Ketogenic Diet For Parkinson's Disease

The low-carb, high-fat nature of the ketogenic diet has drawn interest due to its possible benefits in treating Parkinson's disease symptoms. When the body is in a state of ketosis, which is brought on by the diet, it starts using ketones instead of fats as its primary energy source. The ketogenic diet has demonstrated the potential to reduce motor symptoms and enhance the general quality of life in the context of Parkinson's disease.

The effect that ketones have on mitochondrial activity is one important mechanism underlying the possible advantages. Parkinson's disease is linked to mitochondrial dysfunction, which raises oxidative stress and impairs energy synthesis. Ketones can improve mitochondrial activity and potentially mitigate cellular damage and oxidative stress since they are a more efficient fuel source.

Furthermore, a prevalent aspect of Parkinson's disease is neuroinflammation, which the ketogenic diet may affect. The food may be able to create a neuroprotective environment and decrease the progression of disease by regulating inflammatory responses. Additionally, some research indicates that the ketogenic diet may increase dopamine availability, which is a neurotransmitter that is lacking in Parkinson's disease and may help with motor symptoms.

Even with these encouraging results, it's important to remember that the ketogenic diet is still being studied for Parkinson's disease, and larger, more thorough clinical trials are required to determine the diet's effectiveness and long-term safety. Furthermore, following the diet might be difficult, necessitating careful observation and assistance from medical professionals.

Parkinson's Disease With The Mediterranean Diet

The possible neuroprotective advantages of the Mediterranean diet, which emphasizes a high consumption of fruits, vegetables, whole grains, fish, and olive oil, have been well investigated, even for Parkinson's disease. This dietary pattern is high in omega-3 fatty acids, antioxidants, and anti-inflammatory substances, all of which may help to protect the brain and lower the risk of neurodegenerative diseases.

The Mediterranean diet's emphasis on polyphenols, which have been linked to antioxidant and anti-inflammatory effects, is one of its main features. These substances might aid in the fight against inflammation and oxidative stress, two factors that contribute to Parkinson's disease development. Furthermore, the diet's encouragement of heart-healthy fats, including those in fatty fish and olive oil, can enhance brain function and possibly have an impact on neurotransmitter activity.

According to research, following a Mediterranean diet may help people with Parkinson's disease manage their symptoms and may reduce the chance of getting the disease in the first place. Individual reactions may differ, though, as with any dietary strategy, thus speaking with medical professionals is crucial to guaranteeing nutritional sufficiency and compatibility for every patient.

Additional New Dietary Methods

Apart from the ketogenic and Mediterranean diets, several novel dietary strategies are being investigated for their possible advantages in Parkinson's disease. These include of calorie restriction, supplementing with certain nutrients, and fasting on and off.

Animal research has indicated that intermittent fasting, which alternates between eating and fasting intervals, may have neuroprotective benefits. It might promote the mechanisms that repair cells, lessen inflammation, and strengthen mitochondria. To find out how safe and beneficial it is for use in Parkinson's disease-affected human populations, more research is necessary.

Preclinical research has shown that calorie restriction, a dietary approach that involves consuming fewer calories without becoming malnourished, has neuroprotective effects. It might encourage autophagy, a cellular recycling mechanism that eliminates damaged parts, which could impede the advancement of neurodegenerative diseases. There are currently clinical investigations looking into the viability and effectiveness of caloric restriction in Parkinson's patients.

Numerous substances have also been investigated for their possible neuroprotective properties, including creatine, vitamin E, and coenzyme Q10. Even though some early data points to advantages, more investigation is needed to confirm their significance in the treatment of Parkinson's disease and establish the ideal dosage ranges.

In conclusion, there is hope for people with Parkinson's disease with these new dietary methods; nevertheless, further research is needed to determine the safety and efficacy of these treatments through carefully planned clinical trials. As our knowledge of the intricate interactions between neurodegenerative illnesses and nutrition grows, tailored dietary therapies may become increasingly important in improving the quality of life for Parkinson's patients.

CHAPTER 9

Summary of Typical Supplements for Parkinson's Disease Dietary Support

Parkinson's disease is a neurological condition that mostly impairs movement. Although there is currently no known cure, controlling symptoms and enhancing general well-being can be greatly aided by eating a healthy diet. Numerous dietary supplements have been investigated for possible Parkinson's disease benefits.

1. Coenzyme Q10 (CoQ10): An antioxidant, CoQ10 is essential to cells' ability to produce energy. According to certain research, CoQ10 may decrease the progression of Parkinson's disease and have neuroprotective benefits. Still, the study is being done, and the ideal dosage is still being looked into.

2. Vitamin B6: Vitamin B6 is necessary for the neurological system to operate correctly. It contributes to the synthesis of neurotransmitters, such as dopamine, which is lacking in Parkinson's disease patients. Supplementing with vitamin B6 could be helpful, but taking too much of it can be harmful and worsen symptoms, so moderation is key.

3. Vitamin D: In addition to being essential for healthy bones, vitamin D may have neuroprotective properties. Vitamin D supplements may assist in enhancing muscle function and minimize the risk of falls in people with Parkinson's disease, as these individuals frequently have reduced vitamin D levels. But taking too much vitamin D can have negative consequences as well, which is why customized dosage is important.

4.Omega-3 Fatty Acids: Found in fish oil, omega-3 fatty acids have anti-inflammatory qualities and may help maintain brain function. Although there is conflicting research about the effects of omega-3 supplementation on Parkinson's symptoms, eating a diet high in these fatty acids is widely advised for general health.

<u>**Potential Advantages and Hazards of Nutritional Supplements for Parkinson's Disease**</u>

1. Possible Advantages:

• **Symptom Management:** Certain supplements may help control tremors and stiffness in the muscles, two signs of Parkinson's disease.

• **Neuroprotection:** Certain supplements, such as vitamin D and CoQ10, may have neuroprotective properties that could impede the disease's progression.

• **Better Quality of Life:** People with Parkinson's disease can live better and feel better overall if they eat a healthy diet and take supplements.

2. Dangers and Things to Think About:

• Interaction with drugs: Certain Parkinson's drugs and supplements may interact, reducing the effectiveness of the former or having the opposite effect. Speaking with a healthcare professional is crucial to preventing any problems.

- **Dosage Concerns:** Knowing the right amount of supplements to take is important because taking too much of them can be harmful or cause negative effects.

- **Individual Variability:** Since everyone reacts differently to supplements, individualized strategies for Parkinson's disease diet are required.

Talking with Medical Professionals About Nutrition for Parkinson's Disease

Speaking with medical professionals is crucial due to the intricacy of Parkinson's disease and the possibility of drug and supplement interactions.

1. Tailored Advice:

- Medical History: Before providing supplements, healthcare professionals take into account a patient's medical history, existing prescriptions, and particular symptoms.

- Monitoring: To evaluate the efficacy of supplementing and modify the treatment plan as necessary, routine examinations and monitoring are crucial.

2. Preventing Difficulties:

- Interaction Awareness: By being aware of possible interactions between supplements and Parkinson's drugs, healthcare professionals can prevent problems.

- Dosage Adjustments: Experts are capable of figuring out the right dosage amounts to optimize advantages and reduce hazards.

3. Comprehensive Method:

• **Working Together with Nutritionists:** Working together with nutritionists guarantees a comprehensive strategy for Parkinson's disease nutrition, combining supplements with a balanced diet.

• **Addressing Particular Needs:** Medical professionals can treat particular nutritional shortfalls or difficulties by customizing advice to meet each person's specific requirements.

Incorporating supplements into the dietary management of Parkinson's disease necessitates carefully weighing the advantages and disadvantages of doing so, with an emphasis on the customized advice given by medical specialists. To maximize nutritional assistance and improve overall well-being in people with Parkinson's disease, patients, healthcare professionals, and nutritionists must collaborate and communicate regularly.

CHAPTER 10

Adaptive Cooking Methods for People with Parkinson's Disease

For those suffering from Parkinson's disease, cooking can be a tough activity because of tremors, impaired motor skills, and other symptoms. Patients with Parkinson's disease can preserve their independence in the kitchen by using adaptive cooking techniques, which can greatly improve their cooking experience. Concentrating on order and simplicity is one important strategy. Use pre-cut veggies, select easily handled kitchen tools, and arrange materials in a well-organized way.

Using ergonomic kitchen equipment can have a big impact. Larger-handled devices and utensils that are light and comfortable to hold can help reduce the effects of hand tremors.

Additionally, to lessen the need for hand chopping and stirring, think about utilizing tools like blenders and food processors. These modifications make cooking easier and less taxing on the body, making it a more pleasurable and bearable experience for those with Parkinson's.

It's also very important to modify the cooking environment. Make sure there is enough illumination to improve visibility and lower the chance of accidents. Organize the kitchen such that objects are easily accessible and that there are as few steps as possible between commonly used products. When it comes to kitchen appliances and utensils, contrasting hues can make it easier for people with Parkinson's disease to tell apart different products.

To summarise, adaptive cooking methods for individuals with Parkinson's disease entail streamlining chores, integrating ergonomic appliances, and optimizing the kitchen space to improve safety and effectiveness.

Simple Recipes To Chew And Swallow

Mealtimes can be frustrating and challenging for people with Parkinson's disease since they may have trouble swallowing and chewing. It is vital to concentrate on recipes that are simple to chew and swallow to address these problems.

A key component of developing meals that are appropriate for people with Parkinson's disease is texture adjustment. Choose for easier-to-chew and swallow foods, such as soft fruits, tender meats, and well-cooked veggies. To make items more soft, cook them using techniques like steaming, braising, and slow cooking. Additionally, to make some foods easier to handle for people who have trouble chewing, think about pureeing or blending them.

Adding substances high in moisture can also help make swallowing easier. Soups, stews, and sauces can enhance the flavor and moisture content of food, increasing its palatability and aiding in the swallowing process. Prioritizing nutrient-dense foods is crucial to maintaining the nutritional balance of meals even when they are altered.

In summary, recipes for foods that are simple to chew and swallow require careful thought-out ingredient selection, cooking techniques, and texture to produce satisfying and approachable meals for people with Parkinson's disease.

Organizing Meals for Nutrition and Convenience

Planning meals is an essential part of controlling nutrition for Parkinson's disease, to balance convenience with dietary requirements. Arranging meals ahead of time helps reduce anxiety and guarantee that people with Parkinson's disease have access to wholesome, well-balanced food selections.

Make meal planning easier by putting together a weekly or monthly menu with a range of nutrient-dense items. Make a point of including complete grains, lean meats, vibrant fruits and veggies, and healthy fats. To cut down on the number of time-consuming and labor-intensive cooking sessions, think about batch cooking and storing parts for simple reheating.

Nutrition shouldn't be sacrificed for convenience. Give top priority to foods high in anti-inflammatory and antioxidant qualities, as these can help people with Parkinson's disease. To boost brain function, include omega-3 fatty acids from foods like walnuts, flaxseeds, and seafood.

Meal planning is important, but so is staying hydrated. Consuming enough water can promote general health and assist in managing possible drug side effects. Think about including meals high in water content, such as smoothies, soups, and fruits, in your meal plan.

To ensure a well-rounded and easily accessible approach to regular meals, meal planning for Parkinson's disease nutrition entails strategic consideration of convenience, nutritional value, and hydration.

CHAPTER 11

ASPECTS OF LIFESTYLE APART FROM NUTRITION

The Effect of Exercise on Parkinson's

Exercise is essential for Parkinson's disease management since it has many advantages over just improving physical fitness. Regular physical activity has been shown in studies to improve motor function, reduce symptoms, and improve overall quality of life in people with Parkinson's disease. Walking, cycling, and swimming are examples of aerobic exercises that improve cardiovascular health and release dopamine, a neurotransmitter that is significantly impacted in Parkinson's disease.

Exercise also promotes neuroplasticity, the brain's capacity for self-organization and adaptation. This is especially important for those with Parkinson's disease because the illness causes dopamine-producing neurons to degenerate. Exercises that target different neural pathways, such as balance and strength training, can help compensate for the damage the disease has caused by fostering the formation of new neural pathways.

Exercise relieves non-motor symptoms like despair and anxiety that are frequently associated with Parkinson's disease, even when the physical advantages are obvious. Group exercise's social component fights loneliness and offers emotional support, which helps to manage the illness holistically. As a result, an individualized and regimented exercise program becomes necessary for both physical rehabilitation and a comprehensive approach to improving the general quality of life for Parkinson's patients.

Stress Reduction

A crucial aspect of treating Parkinson's disease is stress management because of the intricate relationship that exists between stress and worsening symptoms.

Stress can exacerbate bradykinesia, tremors, and postural instability, among other motor symptoms. Furthermore, given that prolonged stress has been connected to elevated inflammation, which is a factor linked to neurodegenerative illnesses like Parkinson's, stress may accelerate the course of the illness.

Mind-body practices including yoga, mindfulness, and meditation have demonstrated the potential to lower stress levels in Parkinson's patients. These techniques not only treat the psychological components of stress but also have physiological effects that promote relaxation and may even modify the disease's neurochemical abnormalities. Another useful tool is cognitive-behavioral therapy (CBT), which helps people reframe their perceptions of stresses and provides coping strategies to lessen the impact of these experiences on Parkinson's symptoms.

In addition, support groups and counseling can be extremely important for managing stress since they give Parkinson's patients a forum to talk about their experiences, express their feelings, and get useful advice. Healthcare practitioners might potentially delay the advancement of Parkinson's disease and improve the overall quality of life for individuals with the disease by empowering them to better cope with its challenges by adding stress management techniques into their overall treatment plan.

Best Practices For Parkinson's Patients' Sleep

Parkinson's disease patients frequently experience sleep problems that impair their ability to get enough quality sleep. Maintaining good sleep hygiene becomes essential since sleep disturbances can worsen both motor and non-motor symptoms in addition to making people feel tired during the day. The first step in creating a healthy sleep schedule is to emphasize regular wake and sleep hours to maintain the body's internal clock.

An important aspect of good sleep hygiene is the environment. Reducing light and noise, making sure the mattress and pillows are comfortable, and keeping the room at the ideal temperature are all important steps in creating a cozy and restful sleeping environment. Parkinson's sufferers can greatly enhance the quality of their sleep with these modifications.

Another part of good sleep hygiene for people with Parkinson's disease is managing medication. Addressing nocturnal symptoms and improving sleep continuity can be achieved by closely collaborating with healthcare practitioners to schedule medications optimally. Better sleep can also be achieved by limiting stimulants close to bedtime and introducing relaxation methods like deep breathing exercises into the pre-sleep routine.

To effectively manage Parkinson's disease, sleep abnormalities such as sleep apnea or insomnia must be identified and treated. For the effective identification and treatment of underlying sleep disorders, healthcare experts may suggest sleep tests or other diagnostic assessments. Parkinson's sufferers can maximize their restorative sleep and improve their general health and well-being by emphasizing good sleep hygiene.

CHAPTER 12

OVERCOMING OBSTACLES AND SEEKING EXPERT ADVICE

<u>Managing Nutritional Difficulties</u>

Parkinson's disease (PD) has a profound effect on a person's nutrition and other facets of their life. Managing Parkinson's disease-related dietary difficulties necessitates a thorough comprehension of the symptoms and how they affect eating patterns. The main obstacle is the deterioration of motor skills, which can make it difficult to swallow and chew food properly. Parkinson's patients frequently struggle to stick to a regular meal schedule because of motor changes and side effects from their medications.

Additionally, PD symptoms like stiffness and tremors can make it difficult for people to cook or eat some foods on their own. Dietary changes are therefore required to maintain appropriate nutrition and avoid inadvertent weight loss. To satisfy dietary needs, this can entail changing the texture of food, choosing softer or pureed options, or looking into nutritional supplements.

Managing dietary problems in Parkinson's disease also requires coordinating medication schedules with meal times. It is important to know if certain medications must be taken with or without food to maximize therapeutic effectiveness and reduce adverse effects.

Family members and caregivers are crucial in helping people deal with these difficulties. They must be made aware of the dietary requirements and limitations related to Parkinson's disease to provide a supportive atmosphere in which people with Parkinson's disease can continue to eat a healthy, well-balanced diet.

The Value Of A Multidisciplinary Strategy

Because Parkinson's disease is so complex, treating its many facets—including nutrition—requires a multidisciplinary approach. Creating a comprehensive treatment plan requires teamwork from neurologists, dietitians, physical therapists, and other medical specialists. A multidisciplinary team that takes into account variables including concurrent medical illnesses, medication schedules, and disease stage can evaluate the unique nutritional requirements of people with Parkinson's disease.

Physical therapists can help by creating workouts that improve swallowing and eating motor skills, which will make it simpler for people with Parkinson's disease to deal with food issues. When it comes to modifying drug regimens to treat symptoms like tremors or impaired coordination that could affect eating, neurologists are essential.

Among the multidisciplinary team, dietitians are very important. They can offer individualized nutrition regimens that take into account the dietary preferences, cultural norms, and particular nutritional requirements of each individual. These experts can help people with Parkinson's disease and those who care for them make well-informed decisions about what to eat, how much to eat, and managing their diet in general.

In addition to addressing current nutritional issues, a multidisciplinary approach takes into account the long-term effects of diet on Parkinson's disease progression. It offers a thorough framework that improves the quality of life for people with Parkinson's disease (PD) by acknowledging the connections between the neurological, dietary, and physical components of their health.

Speaking With Dietitians And Medical Professionals

Considering the complex interaction between nutrition and Parkinson's disease, seeking advice from nutritionists and medical professionals is essential to effectively managing the condition. Specialist nutritionists in neurodegenerative diseases can provide customized advice, taking into account the particular difficulties associated with Parkinson's disease.

These experts are capable of performing thorough nutritional evaluations that consider the person's weight, food habits, and any current nutritional deficits. Nutritionists can address the unique dietary issues related to Parkinson's disease through individualized counseling, suggesting changes to guarantee a nutrient-dense and well-balanced diet.

Healthcare providers, such as neurologists and general practitioners, are essential in organizing patient care and promoting communication between various specialties. Timely modifications to treatment plans are made possible by routine check-ups and open contact with healthcare practitioners. This guarantees that nutritional interventions are in line with the overall management of Parkinson's disease.

Consulting with medical experts not only addresses urgent dietary issues but also enables continuous assessment of the person's nutritional condition.

Frequent evaluations can assist in spotting any new problems and enable early actions to stop malnourishment or other consequences linked to dietary difficulties in Parkinson's disease.

28-DAY MEAL PLAN

This meal plan offers delicious and nutritious recipes that are easy to prepare, suitable for beginners, and tailored to promote overall well-being. Each recipe is accompanied by a list of ingredients, directions, prep time, nutritional value, and snack ideas to ensure a balanced and fulfilling diet.

DAY 1

BREAKFAST: BANANA OATMEAL

INGREDIENTS:

- 1 ripe banana
- 1/2 cup rolled oats
- 1 cup almond milk
- 1 tablespoon honey

DIRECTIONS:

1. Mash the banana in a saucepan.

2. Add oats and almond milk. Cook over medium heat until creamy.

3. Sweeten with honey before serving.

PREP TIME: 10 minutes

NUTRITIONAL VALUE: High in fiber and potassium.

SNACK: Apple Slices With Almond Butter

LUNCH: Spinach And Quinoa Salad

INGREDIENTS:

- 2 cups baby spinach
- 1/2 cup cooked quinoa
- 1/4 cup cherry tomatoes, halved
- 1/4 cup diced cucumber
- 2 tablespoons balsamic vinaigrette

DIRECTIONS:

1. Toss all ingredients together in a bowl.

2. Drizzle with balsamic vinaigrette.

PREP TIME: 15 minutes

NUTRITIONAL VALUE: Rich in antioxidants and protein.

SNACK: Greek Yogurt With Mixed Berries.

DINNER: Baked Salmon With Steamed Broccoli

INGREDIENTS:

- 1 salmon fillet

- 1 tablespoon olive oil

- 1 teaspoon lemon juice

- Salt and pepper to taste

- 1 cup broccoli florets

DIRECTIONS:

1. Preheat oven to 375°F (190°C).

2. Place salmon on a baking sheet, drizzle with olive oil and lemon juice, then season with salt and pepper.

3. Bake for 15-20 minutes until cooked through.

4. Steam broccoli until tender.

PREP TIME: 25 minutes

NUTRITIONAL VALUE: High in omega-3 fatty acids and vitamin C.

SNACK: Carrot Sticks With Hummus.

DAY 2

BREAKFAST: Berry Smoothie

INGREDIENTS:

- 1/2 cup mixed berries (strawberries, blueberries, raspberries)

- 1/2 banana

- 1/2 cup Greek yogurt

- 1/2 cup almond milk

- 1 tablespoon honey

DIRECTIONS:

1. Blend all ingredients until smooth.

2. Add more almond milk if needed for desired consistency.

PREP TIME: 5 minutes

NUTRITIONAL VALUE: Packed with antioxidants and probiotics.

SNACK: Rice cakes with peanut butter.

LUNCH: Turkey And Avocado Wrap

INGREDIENTS:

- 1 whole wheat tortilla

- 2 slices turkey breast

- 1/4 avocado, sliced

- Handful of spinach leaves

- 1 tablespoon Greek yogurt

1. Lay tortilla flat and layer with turkey, avocado, spinach, and Greek yogurt.

2. Roll up tightly and slice in half.

PREP TIME: 10 minutes

NUTRITIONAL VALUE: High in protein and healthy fats.

SNACK: Cottage Cheese With Pineapple Chunks.

DINNER: Lentil Vegetable Soup

INGREDIENTS:

- 1 cup lentils

- 4 cups vegetable broth

- 1 onion, diced

- 2 carrots, diced

- 2 celery stalks, diced

- 2 cloves garlic, minced

- 1 teaspoon dried thyme

- Salt and pepper to taste

DIRECTIONS:

1. In a large pot, sauté onion, carrots, celery, and garlic until softened.

2. Add lentils, vegetable broth, thyme, salt, and pepper. Bring to a boil, then simmer for 20-25 minutes until lentils are tender.

3. Serve hot.

PREP TIME: 30 minutes

NUTRITIONAL VALUE: Rich in fiber and essential nutrients.

SNACK: Sliced Cucumber With Tzatziki

DAY 3

BREAKFAST: Greek Yogurt Parfait

INGREDIENTS:

- 1/2 cup Greek yogurt

- 1/4 cup granola

- 1/2 cup mixed berries

DIRECTIONS:

1. Layer Greek yogurt, granola, and berries in a glass.

2. Repeat layers.

PREP TIME: 5 minutes

NUTRITIONAL VALUE: High in protein, fiber, and antioxidants.

SNACK: Trail Mix (Nuts And Dried Fruits).

LUNCH: Chicken Caesar Salad

INGREDIENTS:

- 2 cups romaine lettuce

- 4 oz grilled chicken breast, sliced

- 2 tablespoons grated Parmesan cheese

- 2 tablespoons Caesar dressing

DIRECTIONS:

1. Toss lettuce with Caesar dressing until evenly coated.

2. Top with grilled chicken and Parmesan cheese.

PREP TIME: 15 minutes

NUTRITIONAL VALUE: Protein-packed and rich in vitamins.

SNACK: Sliced bell peppers with guacamole.

DINNER: Vegetable Stir-Fry with Brown Rice

INGREDIENTS:

- 1 cup mixed vegetables (bell peppers, broccoli, carrots, snap peas)

- 1 tablespoon olive oil

- 2 cloves garlic, minced

- 2 tablespoons soy sauce

- 1 cup cooked brown rice

DIRECTIONS:

1. Heat olive oil in a pan, add garlic and stir until fragrant.

2. Add mixed vegetables and stir-fry until tender-crisp.

3. Stir in soy sauce and cooked brown rice. Cook for another 2-3 minutes.

PREP TIME: 20 minutes

NUTRITIONAL VALUE: High in fiber and antioxidants.

SNACK: Edamame.

DAY 4

BREAKFAST: Avocado Toast with Poached Egg

INGREDIENTS:

- 1 slice whole grain bread

- 1/2 avocado, mashed

- 1 poached egg

- Salt and pepper to taste

DIRECTIONS:

1. Toast the bread until golden brown.

2. Spread mashed avocado on top.

3. Top with poached egg and season with salt and pepper.

PREP TIME: 15 minutes

NUTRITIONAL VALUE: Rich in healthy fats and protein.

SNACK: Banana slices with peanut butter.

LUNCH: Tuna Salad Lettuce Wraps

INGREDIENTS:

- 1 can tuna, drained

- 2 tablespoons Greek yogurt

- 1 tablespoon Dijon mustard

- 1 tablespoon lemon juice

- Salt and pepper to taste

- Lettuce leaves for wrapping

DIRECTIONS:

1. In a bowl, mix tuna, Greek yogurt, Dijon mustard, lemon juice, salt, and pepper.

2. Spoon tuna mixture onto lettuce leaves and wrap.

PREP TIME: 10 minutes

NUTRITIONAL VALUE: High in protein and omega-3 fatty acids.

SNACK: Sliced mango with lime.

DINNER: Turkey Meatballs with Zucchini Noodles

INGREDIENTS:

- 1 lb ground turkey

- 1/4 cup breadcrumbs

- 1 egg

- 1/4 cup grated Parmesan cheese

- 1 teaspoon dried oregano

- Salt and pepper to taste

- 2 zucchinis, spiralized

- 1 cup marinara sauce

DIRECTIONS:

1. Preheat oven to 375°F (190°C).

2. In a bowl, combine ground turkey, breadcrumbs, egg, Parmesan cheese, oregano, salt, and pepper. Roll into meatballs.

3. Place meatballs on a baking sheet and bake for 20-25 minutes until cooked through.

4. Heat marinara sauce in a pan and add zucchini noodles. Cook until heated through.

PREP TIME: 30 minutes

NUTRITIONAL VALUE: Low-carb and high in protein.

SNACK: Celery sticks with almond butter.

DAY 5

BREAKFAST: Chia Seed Pudding

INGREDIENTS:

- 2 tablespoons chia seeds

- 1/2 cup almond milk

- 1/2 teaspoon vanilla extract

- 1 tablespoon maple syrup

- Fresh berries for topping

DIRECTIONS:

1. Mix chia seeds, almond milk, vanilla extract, and maple syrup in a bowl.

2. Let sit in the refrigerator for at least 2 hours or overnight until thickened.

3. Top with fresh berries before serving.

PREP TIME: 5 minutes (+ chilling time)

NUTRITIONAL VALUE: Rich in omega-3 fatty acids and fiber.

SNACK: Air-popped popcorn.

LUNCH: Egg Salad Sandwich

INGREDIENTS:

- 2 hard-boiled eggs, chopped

- 2 tablespoons Greek yogurt

- 1 tablespoon Dijon mustard

- 2 slices whole grain bread

- Lettuce leaves and tomato slices for serving

DIRECTIONS:

1. In a bowl, mix chopped eggs, Greek yogurt, and Dijon mustard until well combined.

2. Spread egg salad on bread slices and top with lettuce and tomato.

- **PREP TIME:** 10 minutes

NUTRITIONAL VALUE: High in protein and essential nutrients.

SNACK: Sliced cucumber with cottage cheese.

DINNER: Baked Cod with Roasted Vegetables

INGREDIENTS:

- 2 cod fillets

- 1 tablespoon olive oil

- 1 teaspoon lemon zest

- Salt and pepper to taste

- 1 cup mixed vegetables (bell peppers, cherry tomatoes, zucchini)

DIRECTIONS:

1. Preheat oven to 400°F (200°C).

2. Place cod fillets on a baking sheet, drizzle with olive oil, sprinkle with lemon zest, salt, and pepper.

3. Arrange mixed vegetables around the cod.

4. Bake for 15-20 minutes until fish is cooked through and vegetables are tender.

PREP TIME: 30 minutes

NUTRITIONAL VALUE: High in protein and vitamin C.

SNACK: Sliced Apples With Cinnamon

DAY 6

BREAKFAST: Peanut Butter Banana Smoothie

INGREDIENTS:

- 1 ripe banana

- 1 tablespoon peanut butter

- 1/2 cup Greek yogurt

- 1/2 cup almond milk

- 1 teaspoon honey (optional)

DIRECTIONS:

1. Blend all ingredients until smooth.

2. Add honey if desired for extra sweetness.

PREP TIME: 5 minutes

NUTRITIONAL VALUE: Rich in protein, potassium, and healthy fats.

SNACK: Rice cakes with avocado.

LUNCH: Quinoa Salad with Chickpeas And Feta

INGREDIENTS:

- 1 cup cooked quinoa

- 1/2 cup canned chickpeas, drained and rinsed

- 1/4 cup crumbled feta cheese

- 1/4 cup chopped cucumber

- 1/4 cup diced red bell pepper

- 2 tablespoons lemon juice

- 1 tablespoon olive oil

DIRECTIONS:

1. In a bowl, combine quinoa,

chickpeas, feta cheese, cucumber, and red bell pepper.

  2. Drizzle with lemon juice and olive oil, toss to coat.

PREP TIME: 15 minutes

NUTRITIONAL VALUE: High in protein, fiber, and antioxidants.

SNACK: Greek yogurt with mixed nuts

DINNER: Turkey Chili

INGREDIENTS:

- 1 lb ground turkey

- 1 onion, diced

- 2 cloves garlic, minced

- 1 bell pepper, diced

- 1 can diced tomatoes

- 1 can kidney beans, drained and rinsed

- 2 tablespoons chili powder

- 1 teaspoon cumin

- Salt and pepper to taste

DIRECTIONS:

  1. In a large pot, cook ground turkey, onion, garlic, and bell pepper until turkey is browned and vegetables are softened.

  2. Add diced tomatoes, kidney beans, chili powder, cumin, salt, and pepper. Simmer for 20-25 minutes.

PREP TIME: 30 minutes

NUTRITIONAL VALUE: High in protein and fiber.

SNACK: Baby carrots with hummus

DAY 7

BREAKFAST: Blueberry Pancakes

INGREDIENTS:

- 1 cup whole wheat flour

- 1 tablespoon baking powder

- 1/4 teaspoon salt

- 1 egg

- 1 cup almond milk

- 1 tablespoon maple syrup

- 1/2 cup fresh blueberries

DIRECTIONS:

  1. In a bowl, mix flour, baking powder, and salt.

  2. In another bowl, whisk together egg, almond milk, and maple syrup.

  3. Pour wet ingredients into dry ingredients and stir until just combined. Fold in blueberries.

4. Cook pancakes on a heated and greased skillet until golden brown on both sides.

PREP TIME: 20 minutes

NUTRITIONAL VALUE: High in fiber and antioxidants.

SNACK: Sliced pear with almond butter.

LUNCH: Caprese Salad

INGREDIENTS:

 - 1 large tomato, sliced

 - 1/2 cup fresh mozzarella cheese, sliced

 - Fresh basil leaves

 - 1 tablespoon balsamic glaze

DIRECTIONS:

1. Arrange tomato and mozzarella slices on a plate.

2. Top with fresh basil leaves and drizzle with balsamic glaze.

PREP TIME: 10 minutes

NUTRITIONAL VALUE: Rich in calcium and vitamin C.

SNACK: Whole grain crackers with cheese.

DINNER: Grilled Chicken with Roasted Sweet Potatoes

INGREDIENTS:

 - 2 chicken breasts

 - 1 tablespoon olive oil

 - 1 teaspoon garlic powder

 - 1/2 teaspoon paprika

 - 2 medium sweet potatoes, diced

 - 1 tablespoon rosemary

 - Salt and pepper to taste

DIRECTIONS:

1. Preheat grill to medium-high heat.

2. Rub chicken breasts with olive oil, garlic powder, paprika, salt, and pepper. Grill for 6-8 minutes per side until cooked through.

3. Toss diced sweet potatoes with olive oil, rosemary, salt, and pepper. Roast in the oven at 400°F (200°C) for 20-25 minutes until tender.

PREP TIME: 40 minutes

NUTRITIONAL VALUE: High in protein, vitamin A, and potassium.

SNACK: Mixed berries with yogurt

DAY 8

BREAKFAST: Overnight Oats

INGREDIENTS:

- 1/2 cup rolled oats

- 1/2 cup almond milk

- 1/4 cup Greek yogurt

- 1 tablespoon chia seeds

- 1/2 teaspoon vanilla extract

- 1 tablespoon honey

DIRECTIONS:

1. Mix all ingredients in a jar or bowl.

2. Cover and refrigerate overnight.

3. Stir well before serving and add toppings if desired.

PREP TIME: 5 minutes (+ chilling time)

NUTRITIONAL VALUE: High in fiber and protein.

SNACK: Trail mix (nuts and dried fruits).

LUNCH: Turkey and Avocado Salad

INGREDIENTS:

- 2 cups mixed greens

- 4 oz sliced turkey breast

- 1/4 avocado, sliced

- 1/4 cup cherry tomatoes, halved

- 2 tablespoons balsamic vinaigrette

DIRECTIONS:

1. Arrange mixed greens on a plate.

2. Top with turkey, avocado, and cherry tomatoes.

3. Drizzle with balsamic vinaigrette.

PREP TIME: 10 minutes

NUTRITIONAL VALUE: High in protein, healthy fats, and antioxidants.

SNACK: Carrot Sticks With Hummus

DINNER: Salmon With Asparagus And Quinoa

INGREDIENTS:

- 2 salmon fillets

- 1 tablespoon olive oil

- 1 lemon, sliced

- Salt and pepper to taste

- 1 bunch asparagus, trimmed

- 1 cup cooked quinoa

DIRECTIONS:

1. Preheat oven to 400°F (200°C).

2. Place salmon fillets on a baking sheet, drizzle with olive oil, and season with salt and pepper. Top with lemon slices.

3. Arrange asparagus around the salmon.

4. Bake for 12-15 minutes until salmon is cooked through and asparagus is tender.

5. Serve with cooked quinoa.

- PREP TIME: 25 minutes

NUTRITIONAL VALUE: Rich in omega-3 fatty acids, fiber, and vitamins.

SNACK: Sliced Cucumber With Tzatziki

DAY 9

BREAKFAST: Strawberry Banana Smoothie Bowl

INGREDIENTS:

- 1/2 cup frozen strawberries

- 1/2 banana

- 1/2 cup almond milk

- 1/4 cup Greek yogurt

- Toppings: sliced banana, granola, chia seeds, shredded coconut

DIRECTIONS:

1. Blend frozen strawberries, banana, almond milk, and Greek yogurt until smooth.

2. Pour into a bowl and top with sliced banana, granola, chia seeds, and shredded coconut.

PREP TIME: 5 minutes

NUTRITIONAL VALUE: High in antioxidants, fiber, and probiotics.

SNACK: Rice Cakes With Almond Butter

LUNCH: Lentil Salad With Feta And Mint

INGREDIENTS:

- 1 cup cooked lentils

- 1/4 cup crumbled feta cheese

- 2 tablespoons chopped fresh mint

- 2 tablespoons lemon juice

- 1 tablespoon olive oil

- Salt and pepper to taste

DIRECTIONS:

1. In a bowl, combine cooked lentils, feta cheese, mint, lemon juice, olive oil, salt, and pepper.

2. Toss to combine.

- PREP TIME: 10 minutes

NUTRITIONAL VALUE: High in protein, fiber, and calcium.

SNACK: Greek Yogurt With Mixed Berries

DINNER: Vegetable and Bean Stir-Fry with Brown Rice

INGREDIENTS:

- 1 cup mixed vegetables (bell peppers, broccoli, carrots, snap peas)

- 1/2 cup cooked black beans

- 1 tablespoon olive oil

- 2 cloves garlic, minced

- 2 tablespoons soy sauce

- 1 cup cooked brown rice

DIRECTIONS:

1. Heat olive oil in a pan, add garlic and stir until fragrant.

2. Add mixed vegetables and cooked black beans. Stir-fry until vegetables are tender-crisp.

3. Stir in soy sauce and cooked brown rice. Cook for another 2-3 minutes.

PREP TIME: 20 minutes

NUTRITIONAL VALUE: High in fiber, protein, and essential nutrients.

SNACK: Sliced Apple With Peanut Butter

DAY 10

BREAKFAST: Greek Yogurt With Berries And Almonds

INGREDIENTS:

- 1/2 cup Greek yogurt

- 1/4 cup mixed berries (strawberries, blueberries, raspberries)

- 1 tablespoon sliced almonds

- 1 teaspoon honey (optional)

DIRECTIONS:

1. Spoon Greek yogurt into a bowl.

2. Top with mixed berries, sliced almonds, and drizzle with honey if desired.

PREP TIME: 5 minutes

NUTRITIONAL VALUE: High in protein, antioxidants, and healthy fats.

SNACK: Celery Sticks With Hummus

LUNCH: Chicken And Vegetable Soup

INGREDIENTS:

- 1 tablespoon olive oil

- 1 onion, diced

- 2 carrots, diced

- 2 celery stalks, diced

- 2 cloves garlic, minced

- 4 cups chicken broth

- 1 cup cooked shredded chicken breast

- 1/2 cup cooked quinoa

- Salt and pepper to taste

DIRECTIONS:

1. Heat olive oil in a pot, add onion, carrots, celery, and garlic. Sauté until softened.

2. Add chicken broth, shredded chicken, and cooked quinoa. Simmer for 15-20 minutes.

3. Season with salt and pepper to taste.

PREP TIME: 30 minutes

NUTRITIONAL VALUE: Rich in protein, fiber, and vitamins.

SNACK: Trail mix (nuts and dried fruits).

DINNER: Baked Chicken with Roasted Vegetables

INGREDIENTS:

- 2 chicken breasts

- 1 tablespoon olive oil

- 1 teaspoon dried thyme

- 1/2 teaspoon paprika

- Salt and pepper to taste

- 1 sweet potato, diced

- 1 cup Brussels sprouts, halved

- 1 tablespoon balsamic glaze

DIRECTIONS:

1. Preheat oven to 400°F (200°C).

2. Rub chicken breasts with olive oil, dried thyme, paprika, salt, and pepper. Place on a baking sheet.

3. Toss diced sweet potato and Brussels sprouts with olive oil,

salt, and pepper. Spread on the same baking sheet.

4. Bake for 20-25 minutes until chicken is cooked through and vegetables are tender.

5. Drizzle with balsamic glaze before serving.

PREP TIME: 30 minutes

NUTRITIONAL VALUE: High in protein, fiber, and antioxidants.

SNACK: Sliced cucumber with tzatziki.

DAY 11

BREAKFAST: Spinach And Feta Omelette

INGREDIENTS:

- 2 eggs

- 1 tablespoon milk

- Handful of spinach leaves

- 2 tablespoons crumbled feta cheese

- Salt and pepper to taste

DIRECTIONS:

1. In a bowl, whisk eggs and milk together.

2. Heat a non-stick skillet over medium heat and pour in egg mixture.

3. Add spinach and feta cheese on one side of the omelette.

4. Fold the other side over the filling and cook until set.

5. Season with salt and pepper to taste.

PREP TIME: 10 minutes

NUTRITIONAL VALUE: High in protein, vitamins, and calcium.

SNACK: Sliced apple with almond butter

LUNCH: Quinoa and Black Bean Salad

INGREDIENTS:

- 1 cup cooked quinoa

- 1/2 cup cooked black beans

- 1/4 cup diced red bell pepper

- 1/4 cup corn kernels (fresh or frozen, thawed)

- 2 tablespoons chopped cilantro

- 2 tablespoons lime juice

- 1 tablespoon olive oil

- Salt and pepper to taste

DIRECTIONS:

1. In a bowl, combine quinoa, black beans, red bell pepper, corn, and cilantro.

2. Drizzle with lime juice and olive oil, and season with salt and pepper. Toss to combine.

PREP TIME: 15 minutes

NUTRITIONAL VALUE: High in protein, fiber, and antioxidants.

SNACK: Greek yogurt with mixed nuts.

DINNER: Stir-Fried Tofu With Broccoli And Brown Rice

INGREDIENTS:

- 1 block extra-firm tofu, pressed and cubed

- 2 tablespoons soy sauce

- 1 tablespoon sesame oil

- 2 cloves garlic, minced

- 1 teaspoon grated ginger

- 2 cups broccoli florets

- 1 tablespoon hoisin sauce

- Cooked brown rice for serving

DIRECTIONS:

1. In a bowl, marinate tofu cubes in soy sauce for 10 minutes.

2. Heat sesame oil in a large skillet over medium heat. Add garlic and ginger, stir until fragrant.

3. Add marinated tofu to the skillet and cook until browned on all sides.

4. Add broccoli florets and hoisin sauce, stir-fry until broccoli is tender.

5. Serve with cooked brown rice.

PREP TIME: 30 minutes

NUTRITIONAL VALUE: High in protein, fiber, and essential nutrients.

SNACK: Sliced Pear With Almond Butter

DAY 12

BREAKFAST: Banana Almond Butter Toast

INGREDIENTS:

- 1 slice whole grain bread, toasted

- 1 tablespoon almond butter

- 1/2 banana, sliced

DIRECTIONS:

1. Spread almond butter on toasted bread.

2. Top with sliced banana.

PREP TIME: 5 minutes

NUTRITIONAL VALUE: High in fiber, healthy fats, and potassium.

SNACK: Rice cakes with peanut butter

LUNCH: Mediterranean Chickpea Salad

INGREDIENTS:

- 1 can chickpeas, drained and rinsed

- 1 cucumber, diced

- 1 tomato, diced

- 1/4 cup chopped red onion

- 2 tablespoons chopped fresh parsley

- 2 tablespoons olive oil

- 1 tablespoon lemon juice

- Salt and pepper to taste

DIRECTIONS:

1. In a large bowl, combine chickpeas, cucumber, tomato, red onion, and parsley.

2. Drizzle with olive oil and lemon juice, season with salt and pepper. Toss to combine.

PREP TIME: 15 minutes

NUTRITIONAL VALUE: High in fiber, protein, and antioxidants.

SNACK: Greek Yogurt With Mixed Berries

DINNER: Turkey and Vegetable Stir-Fry

INGREDIENTS:

- 1 lb ground turkey

- 1 tablespoon olive oil

- 1 onion, sliced

- 2 cups mixed vegetables (bell peppers, snap peas, carrots)

- 2 cloves garlic, minced

- 2 tablespoons soy sauce

- Cooked brown rice for serving

DIRECTIONS:

1. Heat olive oil in a large skillet over medium heat. Add ground turkey and cook until browned.

2. Add onion, mixed vegetables, and garlic. Stir-fry until vegetables are tender.

3. Stir in soy sauce and cook for another 2-3 minutes.

4. Serve over cooked brown rice.

PREP TIME: 25 minutes

NUTRITIONAL VALUE: High in protein, fiber, and essential nutrients.

SNACK: Sliced cucumber with hummus

BREAKFAST: Blueberry Banana Baked Oatmeal

INGREDIENTS:

- 1 cup rolled oats

- 1 ripe banana, mashed

- 1/2 cup blueberries

- 1/2 cup almond milk

- 1 egg

- 1 tablespoon maple syrup

- 1/2 teaspoon baking powder

DIRECTIONS:

1. Preheat oven to 375°F (190°C). Grease a baking dish.

2. In a bowl, mix together rolled oats, mashed banana, blueberries, almond milk, egg, maple syrup, and baking powder.

3. Pour mixture into the baking dish and spread evenly.

4. Bake for 25-30 minutes until golden brown and set.

PREP TIME: 10 minutes

NUTRITIONAL VALUE: High in fiber, antioxidants, and vitamins.

SNACK: Greek yogurt with mixed nuts.

LUNCH: Tomato Basil Mozzarella Salad

INGREDIENTS:

- 2 tomatoes, sliced

- 1 ball fresh mozzarella cheese, sliced

- Fresh basil leaves

- 1 tablespoon balsamic glaze

DIRECTIONS:

1. Arrange tomato and mozzarella slices on a plate, alternating with basil leaves.

2. Drizzle with balsamic glaze.

PREP TIME: 10 minutes

NUTRITIONAL VALUE: Rich in calcium, vitamin C, and antioxidants.

SNACK: Sliced Bell Peppers With Hummus

DINNER: Lemon Herb Grilled Salmon

INGREDIENTS:

- 2 salmon fillets

- 2 tablespoons olive oil

- 1 lemon, juiced and zested

- 2 cloves garlic, minced

- 1 teaspoon dried thyme

- Salt and pepper to taste

DIRECTIONS:

1. In a bowl, whisk together olive oil, lemon juice, lemon zest, garlic, thyme, salt, and pepper.

2. Marinate salmon fillets in the mixture for 30 minutes.

3. Preheat grill to medium-high heat. Grill salmon for 5-6 minutes per side until cooked through.

4. Serve with steamed vegetables or a salad.

- **PREP TIME:** 35 minutes (including marinating time)

NUTRITIONAL VALUE: High in omega-3 fatty acids and vitamin D.

SNACK: Apple slices with almond butter.

DAY 14

BREAKFAST: Veggie Egg Muffins

INGREDIENTS:

- 6 eggs

- 1/4 cup diced bell peppers

- 1/4 cup diced tomatoes

- 1/4 cup chopped spinach

- Salt and pepper to taste

DIRECTIONS:

1. Preheat oven to 350°F (175°C). Grease a muffin tin.

2. In a bowl, whisk together eggs, bell peppers, tomatoes, spinach, salt, and pepper.

3. Pour the egg mixture into muffin cups.

4. Bake for 20-25 minutes until set.

PREP TIME: 10 minutes

NUTRITIONAL VALUE: High in protein and vitamins.

SNACK: Greek yogurt with granola

LUNCH: Chickpea and Avocado Salad

INGREDIENTS:

- 1 can chickpeas, drained and rinsed

- 1 avocado, diced

- 1/4 cup diced red onion

- 1/4 cup chopped cilantro

- 2 tablespoons lime juice

- 1 tablespoon olive oil

- Salt and pepper to taste

DIRECTIONS:

1. In a bowl, combine chickpeas, avocado, red onion, and cilantro.

2. Drizzle with lime juice and olive oil, season with salt and pepper. Toss to combine.

PREP TIME: 10 minutes

NUTRITIONAL VALUE: High in fiber, healthy fats, and antioxidants.

SNACK: Sliced cucumber with tzatziki.

DINNER: Turkey Meatloaf with Mashed Cauliflower

INGREDIENTS:

- 1 lb ground turkey

- 1/2 cup breadcrumbs

- 1/4 cup chopped onion

- 1/4 cup chopped bell pepper

- 1 egg

- 1/4 cup ketchup

- 1 teaspoon Worcestershire sauce

- Salt and pepper to taste

- 1 head cauliflower, chopped

DIRECTIONS:

1. Preheat oven to 375°F (190°C). Grease a loaf pan.

2. In a bowl, mix together ground turkey, breadcrumbs, onion, bell pepper, egg, ketchup, Worcestershire sauce, salt, and pepper.

3. Press the mixture into the loaf pan and bake for 45-50 minutes until cooked through.

4. Meanwhile, steam cauliflower until tender. Mash with a potato masher or blend until smooth.

PREP TIME: 20 minutes

NUTRITIONAL VALUE: High in protein, fiber, and vitamins.

SNACK: Apple slices with peanut butter.

DAY 15

BREAKFAST: Banana Walnut Muffins

INGREDIENTS:

- 1 1/2 cups whole wheat flour

- 1/2 cup rolled oats

- 1/2 cup chopped walnuts

- 2 ripe bananas, mashed

- 1/4 cup honey

- 1/4 cup Greek yogurt

- 1/4 cup almond milk

- 1 teaspoon baking powder

- 1/2 teaspoon baking soda

- 1/2 teaspoon cinnamon

DIRECTIONS:

1. Preheat oven to 350°F (175°C). Grease a muffin tin or line with paper liners.

2. In a bowl, mix together flour, oats, walnuts, baking powder, baking soda, and cinnamon.

3. In another bowl, mix mashed bananas, honey, Greek yogurt, and almond milk.

4. Combine wet and dry ingredients until just mixed.

5. Divide the batter into muffin cups and bake for 18-20 minutes until golden brown and a toothpick inserted into the center comes out clean.

PREP TIME: 15 minutes

NUTRITIONAL VALUE: High in fiber, potassium, and healthy fats.

SNACK: Greek Yogurt With Mixed Berries

LUNCH: Quinoa Stuffed Bell Peppers

INGREDIENTS:

- 4 bell peppers, halved and seeds removed

- 1 cup cooked quinoa

- 1 cup black beans, drained and rinsed

- 1 cup corn kernels (fresh or frozen, thawed)

- 1/2 cup diced tomatoes

- 1/4 cup chopped cilantro

- 1 teaspoon cumin

- 1/2 teaspoon chili powder

- Salt and pepper to taste

DIRECTIONS:

1. Preheat oven to 375°F (190°C).

2. In a bowl, mix together cooked quinoa, black beans, corn, tomatoes,

cilantro, cumin, chili powder, salt, and pepper.

3. Fill each bell pepper half with the quinoa mixture.

4. Place stuffed bell peppers on a baking dish and bake for 25-30 minutes until peppers are tender.

PREP TIME: 20 minutes

NUTRITIONAL VALUE: High in protein, fiber, and antioxidants.

SNACK: Carrot Sticks With Hummus

DINNER: Lemon Garlic Shrimp Pasta

INGREDIENTS:

- 8 oz whole wheat pasta

- 1 lb shrimp, peeled and deveined

- 2 tablespoons olive oil

- 3 cloves garlic, minced

- 1 teaspoon lemon zest

- 2 tablespoons lemon juice

- Salt and pepper to taste

- 2 cups spinach

DIRECTIONS:

1. Cook pasta according to package instructions. Drain and set aside.

2. Heat olive oil in a large skillet over medium heat. Add garlic and cook until fragrant.

3. Add shrimp to the skillet and cook until pink, about 2-3 minutes per side.

4. Stir in lemon zest, lemon juice, salt, and pepper.

5. Add cooked pasta and spinach to the skillet, toss until spinach wilts and pasta is coated in the sauce.

PREP TIME: 20 minutes

NUTRITIONAL VALUE: High in protein, fiber, and vitamin C.

SNACK: Sliced apple with almond butter.

DAY 16

BREAKFAST: Spinach And Mushroom Omelette

INGREDIENTS:

- 2 eggs

- 1/4 cup chopped spinach

- 1/4 cup sliced mushrooms

- 2 tablespoons shredded mozzarella cheese

- Salt and pepper to taste

DIRECTIONS:

1. In a bowl, beat eggs and season with salt and pepper.

2. Heat a non-stick skillet over medium heat. Pour in the egg mixture.

3. Once the edges start to set, add spinach, mushrooms, and mozzarella cheese to one half of the omelette.

4. Fold the other half over the filling and cook until the cheese melts and the omelette is cooked through.

PREP TIME: 10 minutes

NUTRITIONAL VALUE: High in protein, vitamins, and minerals.

SNACK: Greek Yogurt With Granola

LUNCH: Lentil Soup

INGREDIENTS:

- 1 tablespoon olive oil

- 1 onion, diced

- 2 carrots, diced

- 2 celery stalks, diced

- 2 cloves garlic, minced

- 1 cup dried lentils

- 4 cups vegetable broth

- 1 teaspoon cumin

- 1/2 teaspoon smoked paprika

- Salt and pepper to taste

DIRECTIONS:

1. Heat olive oil in a large pot over medium heat. Add onion, carrots, celery, and garlic. Cook until softened.

2. Add dried lentils, vegetable broth, cumin, smoked paprika, salt, and pepper. Bring to a boil, then reduce heat and simmer for 25-30 minutes until lentils are tender.

PREP TIME: 15 minutes

NUTRITIONAL VALUE: High in protein, fiber, and iron.

SNACK: Sliced Cucumber With Hummus.

DINNER: Baked Cod with Lemon Herb Sauce

INGREDIENTS:

- 2 cod fillets

- 2 tablespoons olive oil

- 1 lemon, juiced and zested

- 2 cloves garlic, minced

- 1 tablespoon chopped fresh parsley

- Salt and pepper to taste

DIRECTIONS:

1. Preheat oven to 400°F (200°C). Grease a baking dish.

2. In a small bowl, whisk together olive oil, lemon juice, lemon zest, garlic, parsley, salt, and pepper.

3. Place cod fillets in the baking dish and pour the lemon herb sauce over them.

4. Bake for 15-20 minutes until fish is cooked through and flakes easily with a fork.

PREP TIME: 15 minutes

NUTRITIONAL VALUE: High in protein, omega-3 fatty acids, and vitamin C.

SNACK: Sliced Bell Peppers With Hummus

DAY 17

BREAKFAST: Berry Protein Smoothie

INGREDIENTS:

- 1/2 cup mixed berries (strawberries, blueberries, raspberries)

- 1 scoop vanilla protein powder

- 1/2 cup almond milk

- 1 tablespoon almond butter

DIRECTIONS:

1. Blend all ingredients until smooth.

2. Add more almond milk if needed to reach desired consistency.

PREP TIME: 5 minutes

NUTRITIONAL VALUE: High in protein, antioxidants, and healthy fats.

SNACK: Greek yogurt with mixed nuts.

LUNCH: Chicken Caesar Salad

INGREDIENTS:

- 2 cups chopped romaine lettuce

- 4 oz grilled chicken breast, sliced

- 2 tablespoons grated Parmesan cheese

- 2 tablespoons Caesar dressing (homemade or store-bought)

- Croutons (optional)

DIRECTIONS:

1. Arrange romaine lettuce on a plate.

2. Top with sliced grilled chicken, grated Parmesan cheese, and croutons if using.

3. Drizzle with Caesar dressing.

PREP TIME: 10 minutes

NUTRITIONAL VALUE: High in protein, fiber, and calcium.

SNACK: Carrot sticks with hummus.

DINNER: Beef And Vegetable Stir-Fry

INGREDIENTS:

- 1 lb beef sirloin, thinly sliced

- 2 tablespoons soy sauce

- 1 tablespoon sesame oil

- 1 tablespoon cornstarch

- 2 tablespoons olive oil

- 2 cloves garlic, minced

- 1 tablespoon grated ginger

- 2 cups mixed vegetables (bell peppers, broccoli, carrots)

DIRECTIONS:

1. In a bowl, mix together soy sauce, sesame oil, and cornstarch. Add beef slices and marinate for 15 minutes.

2. Heat olive oil in a large skillet over medium-high heat. Add garlic and ginger, stir until fragrant.

3. Add marinated beef and cook until browned.

4. Add mixed vegetables and stir-fry until tender-crisp.

PREP TIME: 25 minutes

NUTRITIONAL VALUE: High in protein, vitamins, and minerals.

SNACK: Sliced Apple With Peanut Butter

BREAKFAST: Spinach and Feta Breakfast Wrap

INGREDIENTS:

- 1 whole wheat tortilla

- 2 eggs, scrambled

- Handful of spinach leaves

- 2 tablespoons crumbled feta cheese

DIRECTIONS:

1. Place scrambled eggs, spinach, and feta cheese on the center of the tortilla.

2. Fold in the sides and roll up tightly.

3. Heat a skillet over medium heat and cook the wrap until golden brown on both sides.

PREP TIME: 10 minutes

NUTRITIONAL VALUE: High in protein, fiber, and calcium.

SNACK: Greek yogurt with granola.

LUNCH: Mediterranean Chickpea Wrap

INGREDIENTS:

- 1 whole wheat wrap

- 1/2 cup hummus

- 1/4 cup chopped cucumber

- 1/4 cup chopped tomatoes

- 1/4 cup sliced olives

- Handful of spinach leaves

DIRECTIONS:

1. Spread hummus evenly over the wrap.

2. Layer cucumber, tomatoes, olives, and spinach on top of the hummus.

3. Roll up the wrap tightly.

PREP TIME: 10 minutes

NUTRITIONAL VALUE: High in fiber, protein, and antioxidants.

SNACK: Sliced Bell Peppers With Hummus

DINNER: Turkey Chili with Cornbread

INGREDIENTS (Chili):

- 1 lb ground turkey

- 1 onion, diced

- 2 cloves garlic, minced

- 1 bell pepper, diced

- 1 can (15 oz) diced tomatoes

- 1 can (15 oz) kidney beans, drained and rinsed

- 1 cup corn kernels (fresh or frozen, thawed)

- 2 tablespoons chili powder

- 1 teaspoon cumin

- Salt and pepper to taste

INGREDIENTS (Cornbread):

- 1 cup cornmeal

- 1 cup whole wheat flour

- 1 tablespoon baking powder

- 1/4 cup honey

- 1 cup almond milk

- 1/4 cup olive oil

- 1 egg

DIRECTIONS (Chili):

1. In a large pot, cook ground turkey over medium heat until browned. Drain excess fat.

2. Add onion, garlic, and bell pepper. Cook until vegetables are softened.

3. Stir in diced tomatoes, kidney beans, corn, chili powder, cumin, salt, and pepper. Simmer for 20-25 minutes.

DIRECTIONS (Cornbread):

1. Preheat oven to 400°F (200°C). Grease a baking dish.

2. In a bowl, mix together cornmeal, whole wheat flour, and baking powder.

3. In another bowl, whisk together honey, almond milk, olive oil, and egg.

4. Pour wet ingredients into dry ingredients and mix until just combined.

5. Pour batter into the baking dish and bake for 20-25 minutes until golden brown.

PREP TIME: 40 minutes

NUTRITIONAL VALUE: High in protein, fiber, and essential nutrients.

SNACK: Greek yogurt with mixed nuts

DAY 19

BREAKFAST: Apple Cinnamon Overnight Oats

INGREDIENTS:

- 1/2 cup rolled oats

- 1/2 cup almond milk

- 1/2 apple, diced

- 1 tablespoon maple syrup

- 1/2 teaspoon cinnamon

DIRECTIONS:

1. In a jar or bowl, combine rolled oats, almond milk, diced apple, maple syrup, and cinnamon.

2. Stir well, cover, and refrigerate overnight.

3. Stir before serving and add more almond milk if desired.

PREP TIME: 5 minutes (+ chilling time)

NUTRITIONAL VALUE: High in fiber, antioxidants, and vitamins.

SNACK: Greek Yogurt With Mixed Berries.

LUNCH: Tuna Salad Stuffed Avocado

INGREDIENTS:

- 1 ripe avocado, halved and pitted

- 1 can (5 oz) tuna, drained

- 1/4 cup diced cucumber

- 1/4 cup diced tomatoes

- 1 tablespoon chopped red onion

- 1 tablespoon lemon juice

- Salt and pepper to taste

DIRECTIONS:

1. In a bowl, mix together tuna, cucumber, tomatoes, red onion, lemon juice, salt, and pepper.

2. Spoon the tuna salad into the avocado halves.

PREP TIME: 10 minutes

NUTRITIONAL VALUE: High in protein, healthy fats, and vitamins.

SNACK: Carrot sticks with hummus.

DINNER: Veggie Stir-Fry With Tofu And Brown Rice

INGREDIENTS:

- 1 block extra-firm tofu, pressed and cubed

- 2 tablespoons soy sauce

- 1 tablespoon sesame oil

- 1 tablespoon cornstarch

- 2 tablespoons olive oil

- 2 cloves garlic, minced

- 1 tablespoon grated ginger

- 2 cups mixed vegetables (bell peppers, broccoli, carrots)

- Cooked brown rice for serving

DIRECTIONS:

1. In a bowl, mix together soy sauce, sesame oil, and cornstarch. Add tofu cubes and toss to coat.

2. Heat olive oil in a large skillet over medium-high heat. Add garlic and ginger, stir until fragrant.

3. Add tofu to the skillet and cook until browned on all sides.

4. Add mixed vegetables and stir-fry until tender-crisp.

5. Serve with cooked brown rice.

- **PREP TIME:** 30 minutes

NUTRITIONAL VALUE: High in protein, fiber, and essential nutrients.

SNACK: Greek yogurt with mixed nuts.

DAY 20

BREAKFAST: Greek Yogurt Parfait

INGREDIENTS:

- 1/2 cup Greek yogurt

- 1/4 cup granola

- 1/4 cup mixed berries (strawberries, blueberries, raspberries)

- 1 tablespoon honey (optional)

DIRECTIONS:

1. Layer Greek yogurt, granola, and mixed berries in a glass or bowl.

2. Drizzle with honey if desired.

PREP TIME: 5 minutes

NUTRITIONAL VALUE: High in protein, fiber, and antioxidants.

SNACK: Sliced Apple With Almond Butter.

INGREDIENTS:

- 2 cups baby spinach leaves

- 1/2 cup cooked quinoa

- 1/4 cup diced cucumber

- 1/4 cup diced tomatoes

- 2 tablespoons crumbled feta cheese

- 1 tablespoon balsamic vinaigrette

DIRECTIONS:

1. In a bowl, combine baby spinach, cooked quinoa, cucumber, tomatoes, and feta cheese.

2. Drizzle with balsamic vinaigrette and toss to combine.

PREP TIME: 10 minutes

NUTRITIONAL VALUE: High in fiber, protein, and calcium.

SNACK: Rice Cakes With Peanut Butter.

DINNER: Vegetable And Chickpea Curry With Brown Rice

INGREDIENTS:

- 1 tablespoon olive oil

- 1 onion, diced

- 2 cloves garlic, minced

- 1 tablespoon grated ginger

- 2 teaspoons curry powder

- 1 can (15 oz) chickpeas, drained and rinsed

- 1 can (14 oz) diced tomatoes

- 1 cup vegetable broth

- 2 cups mixed vegetables (bell peppers, carrots, peas)

- Cooked brown rice for serving

DIRECTIONS:

1. Heat olive oil in a large pot over medium heat. Add onion, garlic, and ginger. Cook until softened.

2. Stir in curry powder and cook for 1 minute until fragrant.

3. Add chickpeas, diced tomatoes, vegetable broth, and mixed vegetables. Simmer for 15-20 minutes until vegetables are tender.

4. Serve over cooked brown rice.

PREP TIME: 30 minutes

NUTRITIONAL VALUE: High in fiber, protein, and antioxidants.

SNACK: Sliced Cucumber With Tzatziki.

BREAKFAST: Peanut Butter Banana Smoothie

INGREDIENTS:

- 1 banana

- 2 tablespoons peanut butter

- 1/2 cup Greek yogurt

- 1/2 cup almond milk

- Handful of spinach leaves (optional)

DIRECTIONS:

1. Blend all ingredients until smooth.

2. Add more almond milk if needed to reach desired consistency.

PREP TIME: 5 minutes

NUTRITIONAL VALUE: High in protein, potassium, and healthy fats.

SNACK: Greek Yogurt With Mixed Berries.

LUNCH: Caprese Salad

INGREDIENTS:

- 2 tomatoes, sliced

- 1 ball fresh mozzarella cheese, sliced

- Fresh basil leaves

- 1 tablespoon balsamic glaze

DIRECTIONS:

1. Arrange tomato and mozzarella slices on a plate, alternating with basil leaves.

2. Drizzle with balsamic glaze.

PREP TIME: 10 minutes

NUTRITIONAL VALUE: Rich in calcium, vitamin C, and antioxidants.

SNACK: Carrot Sticks With Hummus.

DINNER: Grilled Chicken With Roasted Vegetables

INGREDIENTS:

- 2 chicken breasts

- 2 tablespoons olive oil

- 1 teaspoon dried Italian herbs

- Salt and pepper to taste

- Assorted vegetables (zucchini, bell peppers, cherry tomatoes)

DIRECTIONS:

1. Preheat grill to medium-high heat.

2. Rub chicken breasts with olive oil, Italian herbs, salt, and pepper.

3. Grill chicken for 6-7 minutes per side until cooked through.

4. Toss assorted vegetables with olive oil, salt, and pepper. Spread on a baking sheet and roast in the oven at 400°F (200°C) for 20-25 minutes.

PREP TIME: 30 minutes

Day 22

BREAKFAST: Berry Chia Pudding

INGREDIENTS:

- 1/4 cup chia seeds

- 1 cup almond milk

- 1/2 cup mixed berries (strawberries, blueberries, raspberries)

- 1 tablespoon honey (optional)

DIRECTIONS:

1. In a jar or bowl, mix together chia seeds and almond milk.

2. Stir well and refrigerate for at least 2 hours or overnight until thickened.

3. Serve topped with mixed berries and honey if desired.

PREP TIME: 5 minutes (+ chilling time)

NUTRITIONAL VALUE: High in fiber, antioxidants, and omega-3 fatty acids.

NUTRITIONAL VALUE: High in protein, fiber, and essential nutrients.

SNACK: Sliced Apple With Peanut Butter.

SNACK: Greek Yogurt With Granola.

LUNCH: Lentil and Vegetable Soup

INGREDIENTS:

- 1 tablespoon olive oil

- 1 onion, diced

- 2 carrots, diced

- 2 celery stalks, diced

- 2 cloves garlic, minced

- 1 cup dried lentils

- 4 cups vegetable broth

- 1 can (14 oz) diced tomatoes

- 1 teaspoon dried thyme

- Salt and pepper to taste

DIRECTIONS:

1. Heat olive oil in a large pot over medium heat. Add onion, carrots, celery, and garlic. Cook until softened.

2. Add dried lentils, vegetable broth, diced tomatoes, dried thyme, salt, and pepper. Bring to a boil, then reduce heat and simmer for 25-30 minutes until lentils are tender.

PREP TIME: 15 minutes

NUTRITIONAL VALUE: High in protein, fiber, and essential nutrients.

SNACK: Sliced bell peppers with hummus.

DINNER: Baked Salmon With Asparagus

INGREDIENTS:

- 2 salmon fillets

- 2 tablespoons olive oil

- 1 lemon, sliced

- 2 cloves garlic, minced

- Salt and pepper to taste

- 1 bunch asparagus

DIRECTIONS:

1. Preheat oven to 375°F (190°C). Grease a baking dish.

2. Place salmon fillets in the baking dish. Drizzle with olive oil and sprinkle minced garlic over them. Season with salt and pepper. Top with lemon slices.

3. Trim asparagus and arrange around the salmon in the baking dish. Drizzle with olive oil, salt, and pepper.

4. Bake for 12-15 minutes until salmon is cooked through and flakes easily with a fork.

PREP TIME: 20 minutes

NUTRITIONAL VALUE: High in protein, omega-3 fatty acids, and vitamins.

SNACK: Sliced Cucumber With Tzatziki.

DAY 23

BREAKFAST: Veggie Breakfast Burrito

INGREDIENTS:

- 1 whole wheat tortilla

- 2 eggs, scrambled

- 1/4 cup black beans, drained and rinsed

- 1/4 cup diced tomatoes

- 1/4 cup diced avocado

- 2 tablespoons salsa

DIRECTIONS:

1. Heat a skillet over medium heat. Warm the tortilla for about 30 seconds on each side.

2. Fill the tortilla with scrambled eggs, black beans, diced tomatoes, diced avocado, and salsa.

3. Roll up the tortilla tightly.

PREP TIME: 10 minutes

NUTRITIONAL VALUE: High in protein, fiber, and healthy fats.

SNACK: Greek Yogurt With Mixed Berries.

LUNCH: Quinoa And Vegetable Stir-Fry

INGREDIENTS:

- 1 cup cooked quinoa

- 2 tablespoons soy sauce

- 1 tablespoon sesame oil

- 2 cloves garlic, minced

- 1 tablespoon grated ginger

- 2 cups mixed vegetables (bell peppers, snap peas, carrots)

DIRECTIONS:

1. Heat sesame oil in a large skillet over medium-high heat. Add garlic and ginger, stir until fragrant.

2. Add mixed vegetables and stir-fry until tender-crisp.

3. Stir in cooked quinoa and soy sauce. Cook for another 2-3 minutes until heated through.

PREP TIME: 20 minutes

NUTRITIONAL VALUE: High in protein, fiber, and essential nutrients.

SNACK: Rice Cakes With Almond Butter.

DINNER: Turkey And Vegetable Meatballs With Spaghetti Squash

INGREDIENTS (Meatballs):

- 1 lb ground turkey

- 1/4 cup breadcrumbs

- 1/4 cup grated Parmesan cheese

- 1/4 cup chopped parsley

- 1 egg

- 2 cloves garlic, minced

- Salt and pepper to taste

INGREDIENTS (Spaghetti Squash):

- 1 spaghetti squash, halved and seeds removed

- 2 tablespoons olive oil

- Salt and pepper to taste

DIRECTIONS (Meatballs):

1. Preheat oven to 400°F (200°C). Grease a baking sheet.

2. In a bowl, mix together ground turkey, breadcrumbs, Parmesan cheese, parsley, egg, garlic, salt, and pepper.

3. Form the mixture into meatballs and place on the baking sheet.

4. Bake for 20-25 minutes until cooked through.

DIRECTIONS (Spaghetti Squash):

1. Drizzle olive oil over the cut sides of the spaghetti squash. Season with salt and pepper.

2. Place squash halves cut side down on a baking sheet.

3. Bake for 40-45 minutes until tender.

4. Scrape the flesh of the squash with a fork to create spaghetti-like strands.

PREP TIME: 40 minutes

NUTRITIONAL VALUE: High in protein, fiber, and vitamins.

SNACK: Sliced Apple With Peanut Butter.

DAY 24

BREAKFAST: Breakfast Quinoa Bowl

INGREDIENTS:

- 1/2 cup cooked quinoa

- 1/2 cup Greek yogurt

- 1/4 cup mixed berries (strawberries, blueberries, raspberries)

- 1 tablespoon honey

- 1 tablespoon sliced almonds

DIRECTIONS:

1. In a bowl, layer cooked quinoa, Greek yogurt, mixed berries, honey, and sliced almonds.

2. Serve immediately.

PREP TIME: 10 minutes

NUTRITIONAL VALUE: High in protein, fiber, and antioxidants.

SNACK: Greek Yogurt With Granola.

LUNCH: Chickpea Salad Sandwich

INGREDIENTS:

- 1 can (15 oz) chickpeas, drained and rinsed

- 2 tablespoons Greek yogurt

- 1 tablespoon Dijon mustard

- 1 tablespoon lemon juice

- 1/4 cup diced celery

- 1/4 cup diced red onion

- Salt and pepper to taste

- Whole wheat bread slices

- Lettuce leaves

DIRECTIONS:

1. In a bowl, mash chickpeas with a fork.

2. Add Greek yogurt, Dijon mustard, lemon juice, celery, red onion, salt, and pepper. Mix until combined.

3. Spread chickpea mixture onto whole wheat bread slices. Top with lettuce leaves and another slice of bread to make a sandwich.

PREP TIME: 15 minutes

NUTRITIONAL VALUE: High in protein, fiber, and vitamins.

SNACK: Carrot Sticks With Hummus.

DINNER: Baked Chicken with Sweet Potato Mash and Green Beans

INGREDIENTS (Chicken):

- 2 chicken breasts

- 2 tablespoons olive oil

- 1 teaspoon smoked paprika

- 1 teaspoon garlic powder

- Salt and pepper to taste

INGREDIENTS (Sweet Potato Mash):

- 2 sweet potatoes, peeled and cubed

- 2 tablespoons Greek yogurt

- 1 tablespoon olive oil

- Salt and pepper to taste

DIRECTIONS (Chicken):

1. Preheat oven to 400°F (200°C). Grease a baking dish.

2. Rub chicken breasts with olive oil, smoked paprika, garlic powder, salt, and pepper.

3. Place chicken breasts in the baking dish and bake for 20-25 minutes until cooked through.

DIRECTIONS (Sweet Potato Mash):

1. Boil sweet potato cubes in a pot of water until tender, about 15 minutes.

2. Drain and mash sweet potatoes with Greek yogurt, olive oil, salt, and pepper until smooth.

- Serve chicken with sweet potato mash and steamed green beans.

PREP TIME: 40 minutes

NUTRITIONAL VALUE: High in protein, fiber, and vitamins.

SNACK: Sliced Cucumber With Tzatziki.

DAY 25

BREAKFAST: Breakfast Burrito Bowl

INGREDIENTS:

- 1/2 cup cooked quinoa

- 2 eggs, scrambled

- 1/4 cup black beans, drained and rinsed

- 1/4 avocado, sliced

- 2 tablespoons salsa

DIRECTIONS:

1. In a bowl, layer cooked quinoa, scrambled eggs, black beans, avocado slices, and salsa.

2. Serve immediately.

PREP TIME: 15 minutes

NUTRITIONAL VALUE: High in protein, fiber, and healthy fats.

SNACK: Greek Yogurt With Mixed Berries.

LUNCH: Mediterranean Wrap

INGREDIENTS:

- 1 whole wheat wrap

- 2 tablespoons hummus

- 1/4 cup diced cucumber

- 1/4 cup diced tomatoes

- 1/4 cup sliced olives

- Handful of spinach leaves

DIRECTIONS:

1. Spread hummus evenly over the wrap.

2. Layer cucumber, tomatoes, olives, and spinach on top of the hummus.

3. Roll up the wrap tightly.

PREP TIME: 10 minutes

NUTRITIONAL VALUE: High in fiber, protein, and antioxidants.

SNACK: Rice Cakes With Almond Butter.

DINNER: Lemon Herb Grilled Chicken with Roasted Vegetables

INGREDIENTS (Chicken):

- 2 chicken breasts

- 2 tablespoons olive oil

- 1 lemon, juiced and zested

- 2 cloves garlic, minced

- 1 teaspoon dried thyme

- Salt and pepper to taste

INGREDIENTS (Roasted Vegetables):

- Assorted vegetables (bell peppers, zucchini, carrots)

- 2 tablespoons olive oil

- 1 teaspoon Italian seasoning

- Salt and pepper to taste

DIRECTIONS (Chicken):

1. In a bowl, whisk together olive oil, lemon juice, lemon zest, minced garlic, dried thyme, salt, and pepper.

2. Add chicken breasts to the marinade and let sit for at least 30 minutes.

3. Preheat grill to medium-high heat. Grill chicken for 6-7 minutes per side until cooked through.

DIRECTIONS (Roasted Vegetables):

1. Preheat oven to 400°F (200°C). Grease a baking sheet.

2. Cut vegetables into bite-sized pieces and place on the baking sheet.

3. Drizzle with olive oil, sprinkle with Italian seasoning, salt, and pepper. Toss to coat.

4. Roast in the oven for 20-25 minutes until tender.

- Serve grilled chicken with roasted vegetables.

PREP TIME: 45 minutes

NUTRITIONAL VALUE: High in protein, fiber, and essential nutrients.

SNACK: Greek Yogurt With Granola.

BREAKFAST: Avocado Toast with Poached Egg

INGREDIENTS:

- 2 slices whole wheat bread, toasted

- 1 ripe avocado

- 2 eggs

- Salt and pepper to taste

DIRECTIONS:

1. Mash avocado and spread it evenly on toasted bread slices.

2. Poach eggs to your desired doneness and place one on each avocado toast.

3. Season with salt and pepper.

PREP TIME: 15 minutes

NUTRITIONAL VALUE: High in fiber, protein, and healthy fats.

SNACK: Sliced Apple With Almond Butter

LUNCH: Quinoa Salad with Lemon Tahini Dressing

INGREDIENTS:

- 1 cup cooked quinoa

- 1/4 cup diced cucumber

- 1/4 cup diced tomatoes

- 1/4 cup diced bell pepper

- 2 tablespoons chopped fresh parsley

- 2 tablespoons lemon tahini dressing

DIRECTIONS:

1. In a bowl, combine cooked quinoa, diced cucumber, tomatoes, bell pepper, and parsley.

2. Drizzle with lemon tahini dressing and toss to combine.

PREP TIME: 15 minutes

NUTRITIONAL VALUE: High in protein, fiber, and vitamins.

SNACK: Sliced cucumber with hummus.

DINNER: Teriyaki Tofu Stir-Fry with Brown Rice

INGREDIENTS (Tofu):

- 1 block extra-firm tofu, pressed and cubed

- 2 tablespoons soy sauce

- 1 tablespoon sesame oil

- 1 tablespoon cornstarch

INGREDIENTS (Stir-Fry):

- 2 tablespoons olive oil

- 2 cloves garlic, minced

- 1 tablespoon grated ginger

- 2 cups mixed vegetables (broccoli, bell peppers, snap peas)

- 1/4 cup teriyaki sauce

- Cooked brown rice for serving

DIRECTIONS (Tofu):

1. In a bowl, mix together soy sauce, sesame oil, and cornstarch. Add tofu cubes and toss to coat.

2. Heat olive oil in a large skillet over medium-high heat. Add tofu and cook until browned on all sides. Remove from the skillet and set aside.

DIRECTIONS (Stir-Fry):

1. In the same skillet, add more olive oil if needed. Add garlic and ginger, stir until fragrant.

2. Add mixed vegetables and stir-fry until tender-crisp.

3. Return tofu to the skillet and add teriyaki sauce. Stir until everything is evenly coated.

- Serve tofu stir-fry with brown rice.

PREP TIME: 30 minutes

NUTRITIONAL VALUE: High in protein, fiber, and essential nutrients.

SNACK: Greek Yogurt With Mixed Nuts.

DAY 27

BREAKFAST: Banana Nut Overnight Oats

INGREDIENTS:

- 1/2 cup rolled oats

- 1/2 cup almond milk

- 1/2 banana, mashed

- 1 tablespoon chia seeds

- 1 tablespoon chopped walnuts

- 1 tablespoon maple syrup (optional)

DIRECTIONS:

1. In a jar or bowl, combine rolled oats, almond milk, mashed banana,

chia seeds, chopped walnuts, and maple syrup if using.

2. Stir well, cover, and refrigerate overnight.

3. Stir before serving and add more almond milk if needed.

PREP TIME: 5 minutes (+ chilling time)

NUTRITIONAL VALUE: High in fiber, protein, and healthy fats.

SNACK: Greek Yogurt With Mixed Berries.

LUNCH: Greek Chickpea Salad

INGREDIENTS:

- 1 can (15 oz) chickpeas, drained and rinsed

- 1 cucumber, diced

- 1 cup cherry tomatoes, halved

- 1/4 cup diced red onion

- 1/4 cup crumbled feta cheese

- 2 tablespoons chopped fresh parsley

- 2 tablespoons lemon juice

- 2 tablespoons olive oil

- Salt and pepper to taste

DIRECTIONS:

1. In a large bowl, combine chickpeas, cucumber, cherry tomatoes, red onion, feta cheese, and parsley.

2. Drizzle with lemon juice and olive oil. Season with salt and pepper, and toss to combine.

PREP TIME: 15 minutes

NUTRITIONAL VALUE: High in protein, fiber, and vitamins.

SNACK: Sliced Bell Peppers With Hummus.

DINNER: Shrimp And Broccoli Stir-Fry With Quinoa

INGREDIENTS (Shrimp):

- 1 lb shrimp, peeled and deveined

- 2 tablespoons soy sauce

- 1 tablespoon sesame oil

- 1 tablespoon cornstarch

INGREDIENTS (Stir-Fry):

- 2 tablespoons olive oil

- 2 cloves garlic, minced

- 1 tablespoon grated ginger

- 2 cups broccoli florets

- 1 bell pepper, sliced

- 1/4 cup low-sodium chicken broth

- Cooked quinoa for serving

DIRECTIONS (Shrimp):

1. In a bowl, mix together soy sauce, sesame oil, and cornstarch. Add shrimp and toss to coat.

2. Heat olive oil in a large skillet over medium-high heat. Add shrimp and cook until pink and opaque. Remove from skillet and set aside.

DIRECTIONS (Stir-Fry):

1. In the same skillet, add more olive oil if needed. Add garlic and ginger, stir until fragrant.

2. Add broccoli florets and bell pepper slices, stir-fry until tender-crisp.

3. Return cooked shrimp to the skillet, add chicken broth, and stir until heated through.

- Serve shrimp and broccoli stir-fry over cooked quinoa.

PREP TIME: 30 minutes

NUTRITIONAL VALUE: High in protein, fiber, and essential nutrients.

SNACK: Sliced Apple With Almond Butter

DAY 28

BREAKFAST: Spinach And Feta Frittata

INGREDIENTS:

- 6 eggs

- 1/4 cup milk

- 1 cup fresh spinach leaves

- 1/4 cup crumbled feta cheese

- Salt and pepper to taste

DIRECTIONS:

1. Preheat oven to 350°F (175°C).

2. In a bowl, whisk together eggs and milk. Season with salt and pepper.

3. Stir in spinach leaves and feta cheese.

4. Pour the mixture into a greased baking dish.

5. Bake for 20-25 minutes until set and golden brown.

PREP TIME: 15 minutes

NUTRITIONAL VALUE: High in protein, vitamins, and calcium.

INGREDIENTS:

- 2 cups chopped romaine lettuce

- 1 cooked chicken breast, sliced

- 1/4 cup croutons

- 2 tablespoons grated Parmesan cheese

- Caesar dressing

DIRECTIONS:

1. In a large bowl, combine chopped romaine lettuce, sliced chicken breast, croutons, and grated Parmesan cheese.

2. Drizzle with Caesar dressing and toss to coat.

PREP TIME: 10 minutes

NUTRITIONAL VALUE: High in protein, fiber, and calcium.

INGREDIENTS (Beef):

- 1 lb flank steak, thinly sliced

- 2 tablespoons soy sauce

- 1 tablespoon sesame oil

- 1 tablespoon cornstarch

INGREDIENTS (Stir-Fry):

- 2 tablespoons olive oil

- 2 cloves garlic, minced

- 1 tablespoon grated ginger

- 2 cups mixed vegetables (bell peppers, snap peas, carrots)

- 1/4 cup low-sodium beef broth

- Cooked brown rice for serving

DIRECTIONS (Beef):

1. In a bowl, mix together soy sauce, sesame oil, and cornstarch. Add sliced flank steak and toss to coat.

2. Heat olive oil in a large skillet over medium-high heat. Add beef and cook until browned. Remove from skillet and set aside.

DIRECTIONS (Stir-Fry):

1. In the same skillet, add more olive oil if needed. Add garlic and ginger, stir until fragrant.

2. Add mixed vegetables and stir-fry until tender-crisp.

3. Return cooked beef to the skillet, add beef broth, and stir until heated through.

- Serve beef and vegetable stir-fry over cooked brown rice.

PREP TIME: 30 minutes

NUTRITIONAL VALUE: High in protein, fiber, and essential nutrients.

SNACK: Rice Cakes With Almond Butter.

Note: Adjust portion sizes and ingredients according to personal dietary preferences and nutritional needs.

This meal plan is a foundation for a healthier lifestyle. By maintaining these habits, you can continue to support your health and well-being. Thank you for dedicating time and effort to your nutrition. Here's to your continued health and vitality!

SHOPING LIST

PRODUCE

- Avocados (approx. 8)
- Bananas (approx. 8)
- Apples (approx. 14)
- -Berries(blueberries, strawberries, etc. - 8 cups)
- Spinach (10 cups fresh)
- Kale (6 cups fresh)
- Cucumbers (6)
- Cherry tomatoes (8 cups)
- Tomatoes (6)
- Bell peppers (12)
- Carrots (approx. 24)
- Zucchini (8)
- Broccoli (14 cups florets)
- Cauliflower (8 cups florets)
- Sweet potatoes (8)
- Russet potatoes (6)
- Asparagus (2 bunches)
- Green beans (8 cups)
- Brussels sprouts (8 cups)
- Snap peas (8 cups)
- Parsley (2 bunches)
- Cilantro (1 bunch)
- Basil (1 bunch)
- Lemons (10)
- Oranges (4)
- Garlic (6 bulbs)
- Ginger (1 root)
- Red onions (6)
- Yellow onions (8)
- Fresh pineapple (1)

DAIRY

- Eggs (approx. 48)
- Greek yogurt (plain - 14 cups)
- Milk (dairy or plant-based - 4 cups)
- Feta cheese (1 cup)
- Parmesan cheese (1 cup)

- Cottage cheese (4 cups)

PROTEIN

- Chicken breasts (approx. 14)
- Ground turkey (3 lbs)
- Salmon fillets (approx. 8)
- Cod fillets (approx. 8)
- Shrimp (approx. 3 lbs)
- Flank steak (2 lbs)
- Tofu (4 blocks)
- Canned tuna (4 cans)
- Chickpeas (4 cans)
- Lentils (3 cups dry)
- Black beans (3 cans)
- Edamame (4 cups)

GRAINS AND LEGUMES

- Whole wheat bread (2 loaves)
- Whole wheat tortillas (2 packs)
- Rolled oats (6 cups)
- Quinoa (10 cups cooked)
- Brown rice (10 cups cooked)
- Whole grain crackers (2 boxes)
- Rice cakes (1 pack)
- Chia seeds (1 cup)

NUTS AND SEEDS

- Mixed nuts (2 cups)
- Almonds (2 cups)
- Walnuts (2 cups)
- Almond butter (1 jar)
- Peanut butter (1 jar)

CONDIMENTS AND SPICES

- Olive oil (1 large bottle)
- Sesame oil (1 small bottle)
- Soy sauce (1 bottle)
- Teriyaki sauce (1 bottle)
- Italian seasoning (1 jar)
- Dried thyme (1 jar)
- Dried oregano (1 jar)
- Ground cumin (1 jar)
- Ground cinnamon (1 jar)
- Paprika (1 jar)
- Black pepper (1 jar)
- Salt (1 jar)
- Maple syrup (1 bottle)
- Honey (1 bottle)
- Hummus (1 tub)
- Lemon tahini dressing (1 bottle)
- Caesar dressing (1 bottle)
- Tzatziki (1 tub)

BEVERAGES

- Herbal teas (peppermint, chamomile, green tea - 3 boxes)
- Black coffee (1 pack)
- Almond milk (unsweetened - 2 cartons)
- Coconut milk (unsweetened - 1 carton)

MISCELLANEOUS

- Granola (1 box)

- Sliced cheese (for whole grain crackers)

- Freshly squeezed juice (for breakfasts)

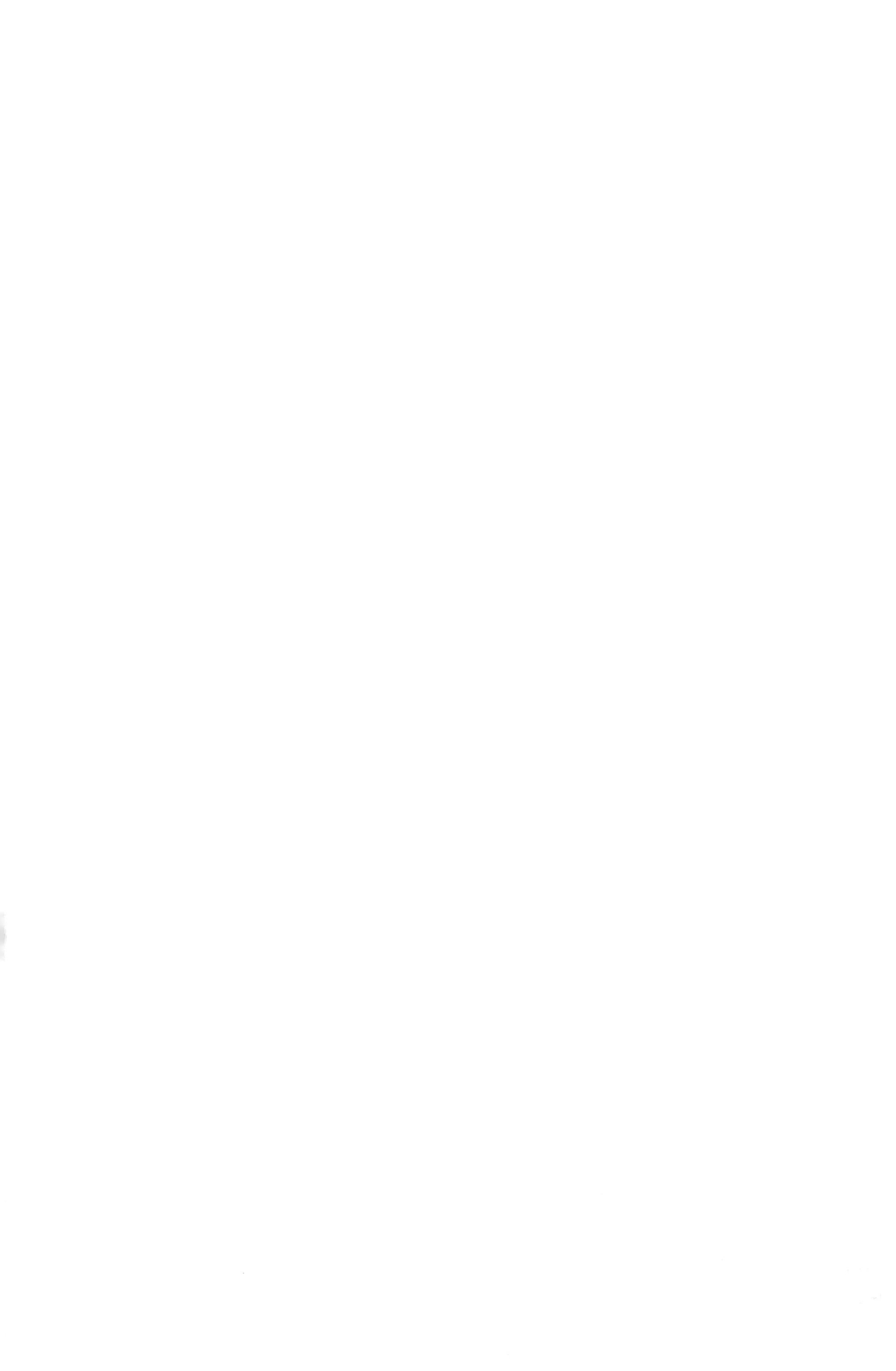